TABLE OF CONTENTS

Top 20 Test Taking Tips

1. Carefully follow all the test registration procedures
2. Know the test directions, duration, topics, question types, how many questions
3. Setup a flexible study schedule at least 3-4 weeks before test day
4. Study during the time of day you are most alert, relaxed, and stress free
5. Maximize your learning style; visual learner use visual study aids, auditory learner use auditory study aids
6. Focus on your weakest knowledge base
7. Find a study partner to review with and help clarify questions
8. Practice, practice, practice
9. Get a good night's sleep; don't try to cram the night before the test
10. Eat a well balanced meal
11. Know the exact physical location of the testing site; drive the route to the site prior to test day
12. Bring a set of ear plugs; the testing center could be noisy
13. Wear comfortable, loose fitting, layered clothing to the testing center; prepare for it to be either cold or hot during the test
14. Bring at least 2 current forms of ID to the testing center
15. Arrive to the test early; be prepared to wait and be patient
16. Eliminate the obviously wrong answer choices, then guess the first remaining choice
17. Pace yourself; don't rush, but keep working and move on if you get stuck
18. Maintain a positive attitude even if the test is going poorly
19. Keep your first answer unless you are positive it is wrong
20. Check your work, don't make a careless mistake

Patient data evaluation and recommendations

Anatomy

Upper and lower airways

The openings to the upper airway are the nose and the mouth. The structures are as follows, nose to nasopharynx, mouth to or pharynx. The nasopharynx and oropharynx form the pharynx in the back of the throat, separated by the soft palate anteriorly. The epiglottis lies at the base of the tongue and it separates the oropharynx and the laryngopharynx/hypopharynx. The trachea is the extension of the larynx. The lower airway begins at the last cartilage of the trachea - the Carina, The carina divides into the right main stem bronchi and the left main stem bronchi. The bronchi divide into lung segments or lobes - two lobes on the LEFT three lobes on the RIGHT. The segments (lobes) divide again into the tertiary bronchi then the terminal bronchioles.

Tertiary bronchioles

The tertiary bronchioles supply the bronchopulmonary segment. The bronchopulmonary segment anatomically divides the lungs, and the tertiary bronchioles lead to alveolar sacs. The alveolar sac is where air exchange takes place. The tertiary bronchioles are conductors. They do not take place in gas exchange. They are important because they contain the anatomical "dead space". When CO_2 needs to be replaced, it is reinhaled from the anatomic dead space. The respiratory zone starts at the division of the terminal bronchioles. When the terminal bronchioles divide, they form the respiratory bronchioles which continue as alveolar ducts. The alveolar ducts are lined with alveolar sacs. The alveolar sacs are covered by capillaries. The respiratory zone comprises most of the lung.

Breathing sounds

The following are descriptions of breathing and breathing sounds:

- Hyperventilation is rapid breathing.
- Crackles are a crisp sound that resembles a fine "breaking", or "cracking" and are the result of fluid.
- Wheeze is a high pitched musical rhonchii. It is heard with asthma or any obstructive airway process.
- Rhonchi are lower in pitch than a wheeze and resemble the sound of a person that is "snoozing". Rhonchi are heard in patients with COPD and bronchitis.
- Rales are moist sounds heard during inspiration. Rales sound like a gurgle because of fluid in the air sacs. Rales are associated with CHF and pneumonia.
- Parenchyma is the functioning part of an organ as opposed to other tissue that acts as organ support or provides connectivity between organs.
- The intercostal space is the soft space felt between the ribs.
- Crepitus is a "cracking" sound that is very dry as opposed to the moist sound of rales. It sounds like rubbing. It is a common sound associated with inflammation and is heard with pleurisy.
- Fremitus is a vibration felt with your hand during breathing, due to obstruction, mucous or tumors in the airways.
- Vesicular breaths are the normal blowing sound of air heard over most of the lung fields. Vesicular breath sounds are soft.
- Tracheal breath sounds are heard when you listen with your stethoscope over the trachea. Tracheal breath sounds are hollow, loud and have a high pitch and loud. They should only be heard over the trachea. Tracheal breath sounds should not be heard in the lung fields.
- Bronchial breath sounds are loud. Bronchial breath sounds resemble tracheal breath sounds and are usually the result of fluid or consolidation such as with pneumonia.

- Bronchovesicular breath sounds are hollow and high pitched. They usually indicate pneumonia or atelectasis. There is a pause heard between inspiration and exhalation.

Proper breathing techniques

Proper breathing technique will strengthen muscles of respiration, help prevent infection, improve oxygenation and decrease dyspnea. Proper breathing decreases the amount of hyperinflation that occurs from air trapping. Several techniques can be taught. Pursed lip breathing acts to keep the airways open for a longer period, improving oxygenation. The patient can breathe easier by taking air in through the nose and then exhales while the lips are pursed. This should be done slowly and in a relaxed environment. Try to get the patient to focus on areas of the body that are tense. Physical relaxation leads to better success. Exercises that engage the diaphragm help the patient breathe more efficiently while strengthening the muscles of inspiration. Have the patient exhale while contracting the abdomen. To strengthen the inspiratory muscles use slow, deep breathing. Gauge the patient's response and stop if fatigue or dyspnea is present. A mouthpiece can be used that have adjustable openings to provide varying degrees of resistance. Encourage the patient to place the hands over the abdomen while watching it rise and fall with each breath.

Physical appearance of comfortable breathing

The patient who is having no respiratory distress breathes twelve to twenty times per minute at rest. The I:E ratio is 1:2. No accessory muscles are used. Accessory muscle use is noted by observing the ribs, and sternocleidomastoid for movement. The abdomen should be moving, not the shoulders. Retraction of the ribs is a sign of increased work of breathing. When the diaphragm is depressed from chronic lung disease abdominal movement is lessened. Paradoxical abdominal chest movement is seen when airway resistance is increased. Look for shallow breathing, fast breathing or slow breathing when assessing your patient. Patients with long inspiratory times may have airway obstruction from edema, inflammation or trauma. The patient with longer than normal expiratory time may have air trapping, trauma or tumor.

Sympathetic nervous system

The sympathetic nervous system is responsible for the release of catecholamine. It is part of the autonomic nervous system. Catecholamine transmits nerve impulse and hormones from cell to cell. The sympathetic nervous system transmits signals to the adrenal gland. When the sympathetic nervous system is stimulated, blood pressure increases, heart rate speeds up, blood vessels in the extremities and mucous membranes constrict and the trachea and bronchi dilate. Patients with bronchospasm require medication to dilate the bronchi. Medications are available that are short or long acting and stimulate the sympathetic nervous system. Common fast acting medications include Albuterol, Proventil and Ventolin. These inhalers are used to provide immediate relief and are administered by way of aerosol. Longer acting sympathomimetics are used to stabilize the patient after the acute problem is resolved. Because these medications are stimulating you should stop treatment if the heart rate increases by more than twenty percent or if blood pressure rises. Recommend a dose reduction. Epinephrine is commonly used to provide relief of laryngeal swelling, control airway bleeding and treat the effects of severe allergic reaction.

Parasympathetic nervous system

The parasympathetic and sympathetic nervous system comprise the autonomic nervous system. The parasympathetic nervous system is normally in control of bodily functions. The sympathetic nervous system kicks in when a crisis is present. The parasympathetic nervous system slows heart rate, lowers blood pressure and dilates blood vessels. Parasympathetic response occurs when vagal nerve stimulation occurs such as excessive coughing or straining. The parasympathetic nervous system can be suppressed to provide relaxation of the smooth muscles. A common medication used to suppress the parasympathetic nervous system is Theophylline (Aminophylline). It is available in tablet form as Theo-Dur. Aminophylline is available for intravenous use and requires blood analysis for measurement of possible toxicity. Combination drugs include Combivent inhaler, Spiriva and Duo Neb. These medications provide sympathetic and parasympathetic effect. Caffeine is listed in the same class of drugs as Aminophylline (xanthenes). It can be used to stimulate breathing in newborns and is given either orally or intravenously.

Leukotrienes

Leukotrienes are chemicals produced by the body's immune cells. They are molecules that are released during an asthma attack or in response to allergens. Medications may be prescribed for your patient that limits the effects of leukotriene for the prevention of asthma attacks. Anti leukotrienes are designed to reduce the amount of leukotriene molecules that that are released. They are for long term management and are not used during acute episodes. Bronchodilators are the medication of choice during episodes of acute respiratory distress. Examples of anti leukotrienes include Singulair, Xolair, Zyflo and Accolate. Review the patient's medication history and ask questions about compliance with medication. Be prepared to suggest the initiation of anti leukotrienes for patients with repeated hospitalizations or worsening asthma symptoms.

Vagal nerve response

The vagal nerve is the tenth cranial nerve. It contains parasympathetic fibers and can lower blood pressure and heart rate when stimulated. The pathway can be mapped downwards from the spinal cord into the carotid sheath, then behind the left bronchus where it forms the pulmonary plexus. During suctioning, coughing from bronchospasm, or episodes of pain or stress, the vagal nerve can become stimulated causing patient symptoms. Look for signs of vagal stimulation during respiratory procedures, especially suctioning. Discontinue suctioning, give oxygen and monitor the patient to make sure vital signs return to normal. Document the patient's response. If a pattern is established, report it to the physician. Measures to minimize vagal response should be taken, such as shorter suctioning time, encouraging deep breathing and using other therapies to keep secretions loosened.

Racial and gender differences

Variances in lung function are seen between men and women, Black, White, Asian, and Hispanic populations. Awareness of this makes clear the importance of entering accurate information regarding the patient's race when providing pulmonary function testing. Though it would be unusual to have to calculate those variables, it is recommended that you become familiar with the following:

For men, [0.148 x height) – .025 x age)] – 4.24

Women: [(0.115 x height) – (.024 x age)] – 2.85

Some deviations from the results are considered standard. For women, the results can deviate within .52 of the considered norm, and for men a deviation of .58 is acceptable. Black persons have less lung capacity that whites, so FVC and TLC values are decreased by 10 -15%. It's been recommended that the Asian and Hispanic population values should be decreased by 20 – 25%. The formula used to calculate the patient's percentage of predicted test results is:

Test result x 100 = % of patient's predicted result.

Pathophysiology

Respiratory alkalosis

Respiratory alkalosis is a state of acid/base imbalance that produces a low CO_2 level, an increase in blood HCO_3 level, and elevated PH. Respiratory alkalosis can be acute or chronic and is caused by alveolar hyperventilation. It is often seen with mechanical ventilation. Other causes are anxiety, infection and fever, central nervous system disorders, drug effect such as aspirin toxicity, or any lung disorder that leads to increased respiratory rate (hyperpnea). Chronic respiratory alkalosis is usually a compensation for metabolic acidosis. The PH returns to normal as the kidneys excrete HCO_3, but the PCO_2 remains lower than normal. Easily recognized symptoms associated with respiratory alkalosis (hyperventilation) include numbness of the hands, feet, or around the mouth, dizziness, shortness of breath and tetany. Tetany occurs due to the disruption in the ionic balance of calcium and is often seen as the patient's hands contract and become painful. As CO2 levels decrease, confusion and fainting can occur. The patient may experience chest pain.

Diagnostic tests for respiratory alkalosis include obtaining a blood gas for analysis and a chest x – ray. Tests may be necessary to determine if there is a central nervous system cause for hyperventilation, such as tumor, or infection. A CT (CAT scan) of the brain, lumbar puncture or MRI of the brain may be ordered. A complete blood count (CBC), urine, blood and sputum cultures should be obtained. Serum electrolytes and liver enzymes will determine if metabolic acidosis is present. The patient is treated by replacing CO2. The patient will need to breathe into a paper bag. As CO2 is rapidly exhaled it will be replaced. It's important to fit the bag tightly around the nose and mouth to provide relief with maximal reinhalation of CO2. PH =7.52 PCO2 = 26 HCO3 = 22 is an example of uncompensated respiratory alkalosis because of the alkaline PH, low PCO2 and normal HCO3. When compensation occurs, the PH will return to normal. PCO2 less than 35 indicates respiratory alkalosis. PH >7.45 indicates alkalosis.

Respiratory acidosis

Respiratory acidosis is a state of acid/base imbalance that causes an increase in CO2, decrease in HCO3 and low PH. Respiratory acidosis can be acute or chronic. It is caused by hypoventilation. Respiratory acidosis is seen acutely in association with asthma, advanced COPD obstructing airflow, medications or substances that depress the central nervous system and neurologic head injury, tumors or neuromuscular disease (Myasthenia Gravis). Respiratory acidosis is seen chronically in association with COPD, congenital deformities of the chest (such as severe kyphosis) severe obesity (Pickwickian syndrome), chronic lung disorders affecting interstitial space (sarcoidosis), and neuromuscular disorders (myasthenia gravis) Often respiratory acidosis is the result of a metabolic imbalance, or combined respiratory/metabolic disorder. Respiratory acidosis causes slow breathing, wheezing, weakness and fatigue, rapid heart rate (tachycardia), confusion, anxiety or restlessness, hypoxemia and shortness of breath. Patients with high levels of CO2 may become somnolent and lose their respiratory drive.

A blood gas analysis and chest x-ray is needed to identify respiratory acidosis. Pulmonary function studies identify restrictive lung disease or neuromuscular disorders. A CT scan of the chest will reveal more information about the presence of pleural effusion, anatomical and vascular abnormalities, tumors, injury or infection. Serum electrolyte analysis will evaluate and allow correction of underlying causes of respiratory acidosis.

The blood gas analysis PH =7.20 PCO2 = 55 HCO3 = 23 is an example of uncompensated respiratory acidosis. It is identified by the acidic PH, high PCO2 and normal HCO3 (the kidneys have not adjusted). PCO2 greater than 45 indicates respiratory acidosis and hypoventilation. HCO3 less than 24meq/L indicates metabolic acidosis.

The blood gas analysis PH =7.40 PCO2 = 65 HCO3 = 35 is an example of compensated respiratory acidosis, because of the normal PH. The kidneys are compensating by holding on to bicarb. (HCO3). The BE (base excess) can also be used to determine compensation. BE = to 0 to +1 or -1 is normal. Use HCO3 or BE to interpret results. When looking at BE, alkalosis would be indicated by BE >0 or +1, acidosis < 0 or < -1.

Metabolic alkalosis

Metabolic alkalosis is a state of imbalance caused by a loss of hydrogen ions, Serum HCO3 levels and BE (base excess) rise. Elevated PCO2 may or may not occur. The PH is high or can be close to normal. Metabolic alkalosis can occur in response to respiratory acidosis and can lead to respiratory arrest. Serum HCO3 >35 is usually the result of metabolic alkalosis. You can also use the BE value to determine metabolic alkalosis. BE greater than 0 - +1 indicates primary or secondary metabolic alkalosis. Hypoventilation, nausea, vomiting, and confusion may be symptoms. It can be caused by diuretic use and excessive loss of body fluids from diarrhea or prolonged vomiting as well as ingestion of alkaline substances such as overuse of antacids. Some general rules to determine metabolic imbalances include observing the PH, HCO3 and BE. Metabolic alkalosis that is uncompensated shows increased PH, HCO3 and BE. Partially compensated metabolic alkalosis will show an increase in all parameters, including oxygen levels. Compensation occurs over time, as the PH returns to normal.

Metabolic acidosis

Metabolic acidosis is a state of imbalance caused by increased production of hydrogen ions, causing a decrease in PH, serum HCO3 and BE, when uncompensated. Metabolic acidosis can be the result of diabetes, alcohol ingestion, kidney failure, or aspirin toxicity. Assessment of metabolic acidosis is determined by the PH of the blood. Compensated metabolic acidosis is reflected by a normal PH. Uncompensated and partially compensated metabolic disorders, (acidosis or alkalosis) are determined by assessing whether the PH, HCO3, and BE are acidic or alkaline. Metabolic acidosis causes rapid breathing (hyperventilation, hyperpnea), confusion and lethargy. The underlying metabolic disorder must be treated to restore balance. Metabolic acidosis is one of the common metabolic disorders that results in hospitalization. It produces rapid respirations by stimulating the chemoreceptors in the medulla. This stimulation in turn leads to compensated respiratory alkalosis from increased alveolar ventilation.

Dyspnea

Cardiac abnormalities can cause dyspnea, such as tachycardia, arrhythmias, valvular problems and congenital abnormalities. Lung disease such as asthma, COPD, emphysema, pulmonary embolism, tumors, cysts, pulmonary fibrosis and sarcoidosis are examples of lung disease that produce dyspnea. Neuromuscular problems such as Guillain - Barre syndrome and Myasthenia Gravis make breathing difficult. Anxiety and panic cause sensations of shortness of breath. Remember that dyspnea is a perceived complaint and is always abnormal when at rest. It is abnormal to have dyspnea when lying flat (orthopnea). Not all patients with lung disorders complain of dyspnea. Identifying the source of subjective complaints of dyspnea requires a complete history, physical exam and diagnostic testing. A chest x-ray, standard spirometry, blood gas analysis and pulse oximetry are basic diagnostic tools. A pulse oximetry is a quick and ready means to assess oxygenation status. Further testing is based on the patient's clinical condition and response to immediate treatment. Use of inhaled bronchodilators and reassessment is often valuable.

Immediate interventions are needed to treat dyspnea, which include reducing the oxygen demand on the patient and providing supplemental oxygen. Protocols in place at your institution must be followed. The patient should be repositioned to a Fowler's or Semi-Fowler's position and re-evaluate. If you can't reposition, side lying with the good lung upwards may help. In newborns with diaphragmatic hernias, this should not be attempted due to possible compression of the chest cavity. Infants with RDS should not be turned in order to avoid compression of the air structures.

The classifications of dyspnea are as follows:
- Class I - The patient feels short of breath with appropriate exertion. Class I is considered normal exertional breathlessness.
- Class II - There may be no subjective complaints of difficulty breathing but the patient is unable to walk an incline or up stairs without symptoms.
- Class III - The patient describes an inability to walk as fast as a normal person without becoming breathless, but is able to walk one mile.
- Class IV - The patient feels short of breath after climbing a flight of stairs or walking 100 yards.
- Class V - Your patient feels short of breath with minimal activity or at rest.

The following is a list of appropriate questions used to evaluate dyspnea:
- When do you become short of breath?
- Can you climb stairs without becoming short of breath? How many?

- Do you have seasonal shortness of breath?
- What makes your shortness of breath improve?
- What makes your shortness of breath worse?
- Can you keep up with others when walking?
- How long does it take you to become short of breath with walking?
- How long do you rest before you can resume exercise?
- Do you experience any shortness of breath at night?
- Are you short of breath when you lie down?
- Do you notice any changes in your breathing throughout the day?

Dyspnea is a person's perception of breathlessness, so targeted questions about how the patient feels are necessary. Remember, that with moderate or severe difficulty breathing it is difficult to speak, so adapt your interview accordingly. Difficulty speaking is an assessment tool in itself.

Breathing disorders

Airway resistance

Airway resistance (Raw) is the term used to describe the difference between inspired air and the amount that actually enters the alveoli. Conditions such as COPD, asthma, emphysema and COPD cause increased upper airway resistance due to a decreased airway diameter. The diameter of the airway determines the amount of resistance. Advanced lung disease results in greater alveolar resistance. Raw score of >8 cm. H2O is considered severe. Airway resistance is calculated by subtracting the alveolar pressure from atmospheric pressure and dividing the result by flow. Measurement is obtained by use of a plethysmograph. The data is recorded, and then calculated during tidal volume breathing. During the test, the patient is asked to breath quickly in order to produce a tidal volume of 500ml. per second. Measurement of air flow helps determine medical treatment. Improved airway resistance indicates the effectiveness of bronchodilator therapy.

RAW is the measurement of the patient's airway resistance. Measurement of airway resistance is performed during mechanical ventilation and in the pulmonary function lab. During pulmonary function testing, tidal volume breathing is performed and the pressure needed to move air in an out of the lungs is calculated against atmospheric pressure. The results are recorded and presented on a graph during a plesythmograph test. Measurement of airway resistance is used to assess the patient's overall status and to measure the effects of medication. It is performed during mechanical ventilation. Normal is 0.6-2.4cm/H20/L/sec. When an endotracheal tube is present, more resistance is added and must be taken into account. Bedside monitoring equipment can be used to calculate airway resistance. To calculate manually, use a manometer and note peak airway pressure after a cycled tidal volume has been delivered. Record the plateau pressure at peak tidal volume, before exhalation. The peak pressure is seen first, and then the plateau pressure is seen. Use the equation:

$$RAW = \frac{\text{peak airway pressure} - \text{plateau pressure}}{\text{Flow} \frac{\text{Liters}}{\text{sec}}}.$$

Orthopnea, radiograph, pulmonary edema, pulmonary infiltrate and hyperinflation

Orthopnea is difficulty breathing when lying down. Ask your patient about orthopnea. Pulmonary edema is an excessive accumulation of fluid in the lungs. It is the result of heart failure or injury to the parenchyma. Pulmonary infiltrate is the presence of fluid (plasma/water) in the lung that occurs when the tissue of the lung is damaged. Hyperinflation is the term used for the presence of air that remains in the alveoli after exhalation. Hyperinflation is commonly seen with COPD/emphysema due a loss of alveolar elasticity. It is also seen in newborns that have aspirated meconium. Pulmonary edema is seen in the lower lung fields and can be present on one side or both. The x-ray shows a white, feathery or fluffy appearance. Pulmonary infiltrate shows a faint white fuzzy appearance. Unless a tension pneumothorax is present on one side, hyperinflation associated with lung disease shows an enlarged hilum, wide intercostal spaces, and clear cut lung fields (from increased lucency). A key finding on x-ray associated with hyperinflation is depression of both hemidiaphragms. The peripheral lung vessels are diminished.

<u>Kussmaul's respiration, ataxic respiration, Cheyne-Stokes respiration, and capillary refill</u>

Kussmaul's respiration is a very deep irregular breathing pattern. It is seen with diabetic ketoacidosis and can be intermittently rapid. The patient's breath may have a fruity odor that can be noted with exhalation. Ataxic respiration is completely irregular. There may be pauses in breathing. Ataxic breathing is a precursor to agonal breathing and is indicative of brain or head injury, tumor or a lesion in the medulla. Cheyne-Stokes respiration is an alternating rapid then slow breathing with periods of apnea. It is seen with congestive heart failure, brain disorders or trauma. Capillary refill is the amount of time it takes the nail beds to regain a pink color after you apply enough pressure to make the nail bed blanch, or turn pale. It should take no more than three seconds to return to normal. It is a quick assessment tool. Delays in capillary refill indicate diminished cardiac output and hypotension; should be noted and documented. Slow capillary refill is likely to produce an inaccurate result when a pulse oximetry device is applied.

<u>Nasal flaring</u>

Nasal flaring is a sign of respiratory distress. When the patient inhales you will see the nares dilating with each inspiration. The nose flares in an effort to reduce airway resistance. Nasal flaring is seen in infants with RDS and in any age group where airway resistance is increased. It is normal after exercise. It should not be seen at rest except in premature infants.

Important terms

The following is a list of respiratory terms:

- Air trapping - the inability to expel gases completely, due to closure of the alveoli.
- Alveoli - the small air sacs located at the end of the respiratory tract, in the respiratory zone and are responsible for the exchange of gases during breathing.
- Anoxia - the absence of oxygen.
- Apnea - the absence of respiration, or the absence of breathing.
- Atelectasis - collapse of the alveoli.

- Bronchospasm - a narrowing of the bronchioles that happens suddenly. It is caused by contraction of the smooth muscles that line the bronchioles and bronchi.
- Croup - inflammation of the upper airway and larynx, causing narrowing of the airway.
- Eupnea - normal breathing.
- Hemothorax - the accumulation of blood between the pleura and the wall of the chest (thorax).
- Hypocapnia - refers to reduced CO_2, caused by hyperventilation.
- Inspiration - the taking in of air, or inhalation by way of stimulation in chemoreceptors in the medulla.
- Stridor - a sound that is high pitched and is heard during breathing. It is the result of difficulty in air exchange and is a medical emergency.

Clubbing of the fingers

Clubbing of the fingers is a seen in patients with long standing COPD and pulmonary disorders such as cancer and sarcoidosis. It is thought to be the result of hypoxia. It can also affect the toes as well as the fingers. A bluish discoloration may be present at the ends of the fingers. The skin is thicker at the ends of the fingers, round, and the ends appearing larger than the rest of the finger. In order to assess for clubbing you should look at the fingers from the side. There will be a noticeable angle from the tip of the finger and the nail. Include this finding as part of your examination.

Peripheral edema

Peripheral edema is usually a sign of congestive heart failure. A weakened heart will pump strong enough to return peripheral fluids to the general circulation. Edema is the result of fluid overload, either from a weakened heart or fluid administration through IV's. Peripheral edema is most common in the ankles and feet when a patient is ambulatory or able to sit up most of the time. Edema becomes "dependent" after periods of prolonged bed rest, and can be found in the back, arms or the abdomen. When assessing your patient, document findings of edema. Edema is measured on a scale of 1 to 3. Record the amount of edema as follows: 1+ = mild edema, 2+ = moderate edema 3+ = severe. To determine the amount of edema, press your fingers into the skin. The more indentation, the worse the edema. When you document, use your scale, i.e. +1/3, or +2+/3. Note the last patient assessment to determine if there has been worsening or improvement.

Pulmonary vascular resistance and shunt studies

Pulmonary vascular resistance (PVR) is an indication of lung compliance. Increased PVR in adults is the result of COPD, primary pulmonary hypertension or as the result of heart, defects that cause left to right shunting (ASD and VSD). Shunt studies can be performed using a pulmonary artery catheter, in order to help determine the presence of a ventilation perfusion mismatch. Shunt is the difference between the amount of blood that is pumped through the heart and the amount that actually takes place in gas exchange.

PEEP can be adjusted and oxygen needs can be determined during mechanical ventilation. Excessive PEEP causes increased PVR. Shunt value should be no more than 5% of CO. The combination of measurements provides information needed for optimal decision making when determining oxygen requirements. Infants who have PPHN or ARDS will display elevated PVR. Increased shunting increases the work of the heart. Over time, increased PVR results in cor pulmonale.

Ventricular fibrillation

Ventricular fibrillation is a medical emergency, requiring immediate treatment. It is accompanied by unconsciousness and absence of pulse. CPR must be started until a defibrillator is available. As soon as possible, defibrillate the patient using ACLS protocol. If you are in the home, call 911. Check the patient for consciousness, check for a pulse, and monitor the patient continuously during CPR and defibrillation. The quicker the heart is defibrillated, the better the chance of regaining a normal heart rhythm.

Ventricular tachycardia

Ventricular tachycardia can result in unconsciousness and low cardiac output. It is treated with Lidocaine unless the patient is unstable. When this happens, synchronized cardioversion is performed. The rate is fast, usually between 110 and 250 bpm.

Atrial arrhythmias

Atrial arrhythmias do not originate as normal, in the SA or sinoatrial node. The impulse for the atrium to contract begins from a different electrical focus. This results in tachycardia. The overall heart rate may not be rapid, but the atrial rate is fast and can be independent of the ventricular rate, except with sinus tachycardia. To diagnose the origin of tachycardia, look at the P wave on the EKG or monitor. A normal P wave indicates sinus tachycardia, abnormal P wave, or absence of P wave means the heart rhythm is not normal. Atrial flutter, atrial fibrillation (AF) and paroxysmal atrial tachycardia (PAT) are examples of atrial arrhythmias. Atrial flutter is regular in rhythm and is diagnosed by looking the EKG or monitor for flutter waves. Atrial fibrillation is irregular and on EKG, no P waves are present. PAT occurs in short bursts and the P waves are different in appearance from the patient's normal rhythm. Sustained episodes of tachycardia can compromise the patient. The clinical presentation of the patient determines the treatment.

PVC's

PVC's are premature ventricular contractions. They may be benign, but in some instances can result in ventricular tachycardia or ventricular fibrillation. They can occur as the result of ischemia. Ventricular fibrillation can follow a PVC that occurs when the ventricle is repolarizing; when the T wave is initiated. PVC's do not always need to be treated. They are considered common in some patients. Low potassium levels can cause PVC's and blood analysis should be considered. Sympathomimetics drugs also cause PVC"S as well as caffeine. If PVC's become frequent, or if the patient is symptomatic, Lidocaine is given to reduce the irritability of the heart. Lidocaine is considered an antiarrhythmic. If the patient is unstable, synchronized cardioversion is performed. In the presence of ventricular fibrillation, unsynchronized cardioversion is used. PVC's are identified by the presence of a wide QRS complex, the absence of P wave and a compensatory pause before the next heartbeat. They can be unifocal or multifocal, that is displayed upward or downward on the EKG. Multifocal PVC's are considered more dangerous than unifocal PVC's.

Sleep apnea

Sleep apnea is the absence of breathing during sleep. Some apneic episodes last up to 60 seconds. The cause can be from a mixed disorder, triggered by the central nervous system in the medulla or by obstruction by the soft tissue. Central sleep apnea can be seen in premature infants (SIDS). Left untreated, it can lead to cardiovascular problems and daytime fatigue. Obstructive sleep apnea is the most common. Alcohol and anxiolytics can cause sleep apnea. People who are overweight and have large necks are prone to sleep apnea. Brain injury such as stroke and neurologic disease can cause sleep apnea. Men are more prone to the disorder. Overnight pulse oximetry, performed in the home or hospital and found to be abnormal is an indication for nocturnal polysomnography. Oximetry alone is sometimes used to provide the diagnosis. The patient's EKG, EEG, oxygen levels and sleep patterns are assessed to help the physician determine the treatment. Obstructive sleep apnea is differentiated from central sleep apnea by the absence of breathing effort seen in central sleep apnea.

CPAP or BiPAP is used to treat obstructive sleep apnea. Thirty episodes of apnea during six hours is guideline used to determine the need for CPAP. The treatment of obstructive sleep apnea depends on the cause. Treatment for narrow nasal passages includes steroid nasal sprays and decongestants. Weight loss is recommended. Dental appliances can be worn to support the soft palate and keep the jaw and tongue from collapsing back. Surgery can be performed to remove tissue from the airway, or support the palate. When CPAP is not tolerated, BiPAP can be tried. BiPAP allows less resistance during exhalation and is more comfortable for the patient. Newer CPAP machines are available that will automatically titrate CPAP. Central sleep apnea may require tracheostomy or intubation. Mixed sleep apnea requires a combination of the therapies discussed.

Bronchopulmonary dysplasia

Bronchopulmonary dysplasia is pulmonary dysfunction that is the result of abnormal growth of the lung tissue and pulmonary vasculature. It most commonly develops in preterm neonates who have received prolonged mechanical ventilation and/or high levels of oxygen. It can also develop in full term neonates who experience respiratory problems, and has been seen in adults. It usually occurs as the result of RDS. BPD can be avoided by minimizing mean airway pressures and high oxygen flow during mechanical ventilation. Wean from the ventilator quickly. Maintain Pao2 levels at 60-70torr in the neonate. Medications are used to prevent inflammation and fluid buildup. Common medications include Theophylline, Lasix and Dexamethasone. Replacement of surfactant in RDS is given to minimize the possibility of BPD. During mechanical ventilation, changes in airway pressure (Paw) are monitored. Decreased lung compliance or increased airway pressure will result in an increase in mean airway pressure. This increase in the mean airway pressure is thought to damage the lungs (more than 12cm/H20). Improvement in lung function is evident by reductions in mean airway pressure.

MI

Symptoms of Myocardial infarction (MI) can be varied and are not limited to just chest pain. Usually pain is located midsternally and can radiate down the left arm or to the jaw. Sometimes chest discomfort is the only complaint. A feeling of heaviness may be present, or pressure in the chest. Abdominal pain or epigastric pain can be seen. The patient may complain of nausea and become diaphoretic. Shortness of breath may or may not occur. An EKG is needed to determine if acute changes are present. Specific EKG changes determine cardiac ischemia or acute myocardial infarction. Typical EKG changes include elevation of the ST segments. Ischemia is evidence by ST segment depression. If your patient is complaining of chest pain it should always be documented and further investigated. Provide oxygen by nasal cannula at 2L/min. Monitor the patient's heart rate and rhythm. Blood samples are needed to check cardiac troponin levels.

Lung consolidation and pleural fluid

Lung consolidation occurs when alveoli are filled with fluid. It is usually isolation in one lung segment. The alveoli segment can fill with fluid from blood, aspiration, inflammation from pneumonia or inflammatory type cells. Pleural fluid is evidenced on chest radiograph when blunting occurs at the costophrenic angle. Look for pleural fluid in the lower lungs or in the intrapleural space. The physician may request a lateral decubitus view of the chest to look for smaller fluid levels as it shifts when the patient's position is changed. The accumulation of fluid in the pleural or intrapleural space can be the result of pneumonia, tumors or congestive heart failure. Injury to the chest can cause internal bleeding that leads to hemothorax. The chest x-ray shows a white shadow when consolidation is present. The shadow is an indication that air is absent and fluid has entered the alveoli.

Pulmonary embolism

Pulmonary embolism occurs when a clot or thrombus has developed in the venous circulation and the clot becomes mobilized. It can travel to the pulmonary blood vessels and cause sudden symptoms and measurable changes in the patient's pulmonary function. Often the symptoms are vague. Many clinicians feel that the diagnosis of pulmonary embolism should be ruled out for any patient with chest pain that has an undetermined cause. Symptoms include shortness of breath and chest pain. Hemoptysis can occur.

Massive pulmonary emboli can cause death. You should be aware that pulmonary embolism is a frequent occurrence post trauma to the extremities and during prolonged bed rest.

Atelectasis and infiltrates may be seen on chest radiograph over time. The patient's respiratory rate may increase. When pulmonary embolism is present the amount of dead space increases. To perform the Vd/Vt test: $Vd/Vt = (PaCO2 - PECO2)\ PaCO2$. Normal values are 0.20–0.40. Review other causes of increased dead space. If the patient is at risk for pulmonary embolism the respiratory therapist should recommend further studies.

Patient Data

Patient history

Reviewing a patient chart includes reviewing the admission history, physical and demographic sheet; noting what symptoms your patient had on admission and comparing with the present symptoms; reviewing the physician's progress notes and orders as well as the respiratory therapy and nurse's notes. The acuity of the patient should be determined. It must be decided if your patient is acutely ill, in a state of crisis, getting progressively worse, has repeated bouts of the same illness, or has multiple problems. After obtaining a brief reassessment, treatment should be provided. Acute illness includes trauma, MI (heart attack), choking or aspiration, severe types of pneumonia, pulmonary embolism and pneumothorax. Examples of repeated illness include asthma, CHF, angina, and neuromuscular diseases. Multiple illnesses include metabolic disorders kidney failure, infections, and chronic pulmonary disease, pulmonary fibrosis cystic fibrosis. Patients who are getting progressively worse fall into the intermittent or multiple problem categories. They are usually persons with long standing COPD, kidney disease, infections, pneumonia and neuromuscular disease. Clarification from the physician should be sought whenever orders are unclear. Orders must be signed by the physician and the date checked. The patient's name must be on the order sheet and it should be checked for accuracy.

Cardiopulmonary system measurements

Heart rate

The patient's heart rate can be palpated at the carotid artery, brachial artery, radial artery, femoral artery or at the apex of the heart. It is most easily heard at the left intercostal space, mid clavicle. This is where the point of maximum impulse lies (PMI). Irregular heart rates are normal in infants and young people. Listen for one full minute to accurately measure an irregular heart rate. A weak pulse usually means low blood pressure or decreased cardiac output. A strong, bounding pulse can indicate high blood pressure. Normal resting heart rate is based on age: Adults: 60-100bpm, 4yrs. 70-115, 3yrs. 80-120 1-2yrs. 80-140 and infants 70-170. Variances are allowed for increased oxygen demands, as with any exertion.

Heart rhythm

Heart rate normally increases with inspiration due to negative intrathoracic pressure. Increased and sudden heart rate irregularities are abnormal. When monitoring your patient during treatment, note and document any changes in heart rate and rhythm. Listen to the heart rhythm with your stethoscope. If you are providing a treatment and observe an abnormality, discontinue the treatment until the patient is evaluated. Recommend an EKG if you observe any abnormal heart sounds. If you cannot hear any heart sounds, assess for cardiac arrest and start resuscitation. Premature ventricular contractions (PVC's) can be heard with the stethoscope. You will hear a pause (compensatory pause) that follows a premature beat. Atrial fibrillation, paroxysmal atrial tachycardia, atrioventricular block and premature atrial contractions (PAC's) are examples of irregular heart rhythms. It is not possible to determine the origin of irregular heart rates without obtaining an EKG.

Blood pressure measurements

Normal range of blood pressures is <120/80 in adults and >60-100/20-70 for infants. Blood pressure is measured in mm. of mercury – mm/hg.   Obtain a baseline blood pressure on admission. Blood pressure readings vary, depending on the disease process. Blood pressure values are reflective of the health of the left ventricle of the heart. It is the sum of the heart rate and stroke volume, elasticity of the arteries and the amount of circulating blood volume. Increased heart rates are the body's attempt to raise blood pressure. Hypertension is considered present if the systolic blood pressure is greater than 140/90. Hypotension exists when blood pressure is less than 80 systolic. Many factors influence blood pressure. Pain, exertion and anxiety can raise blood pressure.

External chest examination

The following are the steps in an external chest examination:
- Look for outward signs of dyspnea such as the use of accessory muscles and chest deformities.
- Check the trachea for midline position.
- Examine the chest with the patient undressed or wearing a hospital gown. Press on the ribs and the sternal area to identify any painful areas.
- Check the chest for equal expansion.
- Palpate for fremitus.
- Percuss the chest for dullness or increased resonance.

The diaphragm of the stethoscope is used to listen to the lungs, the bell of the stethoscope is used to listen to the heart .Start at the top and work to the lung bases from side to side. Note the breath sounds in each lung field. Have the patient breathe slowly, through the mouth. Never listen through clothing. When you have completed your assessment document your findings; include the date and time.

Sputum production

When assessing sputum production, question the patient about the presence of a cough. Is the cough productive or non productive? When is sputum expectorated (morning or evening, at work)? Exposure to allergens, smoking and foods can produce sputum. Find out if there are seasonal changes in sputum production to determine if allergies are contributing to the patient's respiratory problems. Ask the patient if it is easy to cough up sputum. Ask for descriptions such "thick, thin or watery". Document your discussion. Provide aerosol treatments in an effective manner. Hand held nebulizer, inhalers with pre measured dosing and IPPB are effective. IPPB may be the preferred method if a patient is unconscious, very weak or unable to cooperate. IPPB can also be used in the home setting.

Fluid balance (I +O)

Intake of fluids and total fluid outputs should normally be equal over a 24 hr. period. Patients who are hospitalized show marked imbalances that require assessment. The intake of fluids includes those ingested orally, by way of nasogastric or other feeding tubes and intravenous fluid. Fluid output comes from urination, nasogastric, chest tube, and wound drainage devices. Vomiting and diarrhea contribute to the body's loss of fluid. Diaphoresis accounts for insensible loss of fluids. Newborns lose body fluid when the environment is less than 1 degree of body temperature. Humidified oxygen helps balance insensible fluid loss. Critically ill patients require close monitoring of intake and output. Imbalances can cause tachycardia, hypotension, hypertension or volume overload, depending on the imbalance. All intake and output is normally measured after eight hours. Patients with dehydration have a low urinary output, low pulmonary wedge pressure, confusion and low central venous pressure. Overly hydrated patients, especially those with renal failure may also have low urinary output, but can become overloaded with fluid volume, leading to pulmonary edema.

Cardiac output

Cardiac output is measured with a special (thermodilution port) of a Swan Ganz catheter. Cardiac output defines the ability of the heart to pump properly and provide the organs of with necessary oxygen and nutrients. Cardiac output is the result of heart rate x SV (stroke volume).

SV

Stroke volume (SV) is the amount of blood ejected by the heart during one contraction of the left ventricle.

SVR

Systemic vascular resistance (SVR) is the amount of resistance produced by the blood vessels when blood is circulated through the vascular beds. It includes all of the blood vessels, including the pulmonary vasculature. It is affected by circulating volume and the diameter of the blood vessels. SVR is the result of blood pressure divided by cardiac output.

Normal values and definitions

<u>CO</u>

Cardiac output (CO) norms vary somewhat. Normal adult CO, at rest is 4-8 liters/min. Infants normally have a CO output of 0.6-0.8 liters/min. High CO output is seen when oxygen demands increase/ higher outputs are normal with exercise. In the critically ill patient, high outputs may be associated with fever and increased oxygen demands, due to changes in cardiopulmonary function. Low CO is the result of heart failure, low circulating volume and increased peripheral vascular resistance. Low CO is present with hypotension.

SVR

Normal SVR for adults is 15-20 mm/Hg. SVR increases and decreases with vasoconstriction and vasodilatation. When measured in dynes, the normal is between 900 and 1400 dynes/sec/cm. (-5).

CI

Cardiac index (CI) measurements fall within normal parameters when correlated with body surface area. Larger adults will have greater CO as well as a higher CI. A chart is used to calculate BSA (body surface area) and the normal results are reflected when BSA is factored into the calculation. Low or high cardiac index follows the same causes and necessary treatments as does low or high cardiac output.

PAO2

PAO2 is the partial pressure of oxygen in the alveoli.

PH2O

PH2O is the pressure exerted by the presence of water vapor in the lungs. PH2O is affected by body temperature and it increases with higher temperatures and decreases if body temperature is below normal (hypothermia).

FIO2

FIO2 is the percentage of inspired oxygen, the fractional concentration of oxygen.

PaO2

PaO2 is the symbol used when arterial oxygen is measured.

Reflective oximetry

Reflective oximetry makes use of light transmission. A quadruple lumen pulmonary artery catheter is used. Oxyhemoglobin measurements can then be continuously measured and displayed on the monitor. The quadruple lumen catheter has other functions and is used to measure PAP, PVO2 and other pulmonary and cardiac calculations similar to those performed with other pulmonary artery catheters. A fiberoptic bundle is present in the quadruple lumen catheter to take measurements of blood as it circulates through the pulmonary artery. In this way, SVO2 can be measured and mixed venous blood samples can be obtained. SVO2 measurement provides an indication of the amount of oxygen consumption. In low cardiac output states, SVO2 is reduced. Medication may be needed to increase cardiac output. Increased oxygenation is required. Reflective oximetry results less than 30 torr are indicative of hypoxemia.

Six minute walk

Asses a patient by performing the six minute walk. Have the patient walk as far as they can during this time frame. The six minute walk test is believed to be a good overall predictor of mortality. A patient who cannot walk at least 200 yards in six minutes is believed to have a greater risk of six month mortality. Explain the procedure to the patient. Assess and document the vital signs and pulse oximetry reading and monitor the patient during the walk. Assess and record vital signs and oxygen levels at the end of the walk. If needed, let the patient rest during the walk. After six minutes the total distance walked is measured. Record the patient's perception of dyspnea. The patient should perform the test in a completely independent fashion with no help from the family or therapist. Supplemental oxygen devices should be managed by the patient in order to fully assess how the patient can adapt in the home. Use the six minute walk results for setting goals and repeat it as the patient progresses.

Changes in respiratory rate

The patient's respiratory rate may need to be adjusted during mechanical ventilation when the tidal volume cannot be adjusted. In general, higher respiratory rates produce lower CO_2 levels. Respiratory rates and tidal volumes are initially estimated based on the patient's weight. After the initial rate is established, as above, blood gas analysis is performed. A new respiratory rate may need to be calculated to bring the patient's CO2 values back into range. The formula is the same formula used to calculate tidal volume changes. In the first equation, the values are current. In the second equation the rate and PCO2 are those that are desired.*

$$(VT - [anatomic\ VD + mechanical\ VD]) \times f \times PCO2 =$$
$$(VT - [anatomic\ VD + mechanical\ VD]) \times f^* \times PCO2^*$$

Pulse oximetry

The pulse oximetry measures the oxygen saturation in the blood by use of a spectrophotometer. The light or spectrophotometer is able to detect hemoglobin in the arterial blood that is saturated with oxygen. The pulse oximeter can be attached to the earlobe or finger, but it has to be aligned properly and secure to display and accurate reading. Accurate readings are dependent on a strong pulse wave. The pulse wave is displayed on the oximetry monitor. When oxygen saturations drop to less than 70% readings become inaccurate. When poor perfusion is an issue, the oximeter will display incorrect readings. Nail polish and acrylic nails must be removed in order for the spectrophotometer to be able to correctly sense. Always investigate the cause of low pulse oximetry readings. Remember that CO2 abnormalities are separately monitored. In addition, remember that in the presence of carbon monoxide inhalation the pulse oximeter is of no value with regards to true oxygen saturation levels.

Lab Data

Serum electrolytes

Serum electrolytes include Potassium (K), Chloride (CL), CO2, Sodium (NA), HCO3 (bicarb), Calcium (CA), Glucose (GL or BS). Normal values can vary slightly depending on the regional laboratory references. All patients who are admitted to the hospital will receive a serum electrolyte panel. Ongoing testing is necessary to monitor the effects of medication and medical interventions. Abnormalities need to be corrected as soon as possible to facilitate optimal cellular function. Other tests that are normally evaluated on admission are CBC (complete blood count), urinalysis and clotting studies (coagulation). If infection is suspected, cultures of sputum and blood may be obtained. Various X-Ray results may also be available. Remember to review all of your patient's lab tests. Normal electrolyte values are:

- Chloride (CL)   95 - 106
- Sodium (Na)   135 -145
- Bicarb (HCO3)   22 - 25
- Calcium (Ca)   4.5 - 5.5
- Potassium (K)   3.5 - 5.5
- Glucose   70 - 110

Serum potassium

Low or high levels of serum potassium interfere with nerve conduction. Potassium abnormalities can cause a variety of symptoms. High potassium, or hyperkalemia causes EKG changes, muscle weakness and heart rhythm disturbances and are associated with kidney disease and certain medications that cause the body to retain potassium. Low potassium, hypokalemia, causes EKG changes, muscle weakness, muscle aches, produces low sodium levels, seizures, and can be life threatening. The most common cause of low potassium is the use of diuretics. Poor intake of potassium rich foods and diabetic ketoacidosis are other causes. Hypokalemia produces metabolic alkalosis.

Abnormal amounts of potassium in the blood are reflected by distinct EKG changes. Be prepared to recommend potassium replacement if you notice signs of hypokalemia (low potassium) on EKG. Hypokalemia causes feelings of palpitations, or irregular heart rate and this is displayed as skipped or premature beats on the EKG. The presence of U waves is a classic EKG change when potassium in the body is depleted. Normal EKG displays a P wave, QRS complex, followed by a T wave. When potassium levels are low the T wave is followed by another wave, the U wave, rather than returning to baseline. The EKG must be of good quality so as not to mistake interference with an EKG abnormality. Normally rounded T waves become flattened, ST depression may be seen and the QT interval may be longer than normal. Hyperkalemic EKG changes show T waves changes that are peaked and high. Slow heart rate (bradycardia) may accompany hyperkalemia. The QRS complex will appear wider than normal. Potassium is one of the most important electrolytes to monitor when providing patient care.

Serum chloride

Chlorides help control the body's acid base balance and work in conjunction with sodium to regulate balance. Low chloride or high chloride levels may be caused by certain medications. High levels, hyperchloremia, can occur with dehydration, metabolic acidosis, and respiratory alkalosis. Low levels, hypochloremia can occur with congestive heart failure, chronic respiratory acidosis (compensated), metabolic alkalosis, overhydration, and kidney disorders.

Serum CO2 and sodium

CO_2 in the serum is really a measurement of serum HCO_3. Most CO_2 in the blood is in the form of HCO_3. A serum CO_2 level is usually a part of the electrolyte tests ordered in the hospital. Abnormalities are reflection of fluid loss or retention. Low levels can mean aspirin toxicity or metabolic acidosis. High levels can be the result of hyperaldosteronism, respiratory disorders, excessive vomiting or Cushing's syndrome.

Sodium helps maintain normal blood pressure and regulates how body fluids are held or eliminated by the body. Sodium is needed to regulate the heart and for proper nerve conduction. High sodium levels (hypernatremia) cause confusion, lethargy, fatigue, restlessness and coma from brain swelling. Hypernatremia can be caused by dehydration (water deficit in the body from fluid loss), diuretic use, diabetes insipidus and Cushing's syndrome. Symptoms are lethargy, swelling, seizures and coma. Hyponatremia (low sodium) can be the result of hormonal imbalance (Addison's disease, hypothyroidism), diuretics, chronic vomiting or diarrhea, certain medications and kidney problems. Symptoms include confusion, headache, no appetite, irritability, muscle weakness and cramps.

HCO3, calcium and glucose

The body retains HCO3 to adjust for respiratory acidosis when the PCO2 is elevated. A decreased PCO2 levels causes the kidneys to eliminate Bicarb. This in turn regulates the effects of respiratory alkalosis.

Calcium controls neuromuscular function and nerve conduction. Low calcium (hypocalcemia) causes twitching and excessive nerve response to stimulation. Common causes of hypocalcemia are hormonal disorders (hypoparathyroid), vitamin D deficiency, pancreatitis, and kidney failure. High calcium (hypercalcemia) causes lethargy and muscle weakness. Common causes of hypocalcemia are hyperparathyroidism, too much vitamin D, bone cancer, and sarcoidosis.

Glucose regulates energy in the body. Imbalance causes a cascade of respiratory, neurologic and metabolic abnormalities .High glucose (hyperglycemia) can be caused by diabetes, Cushing's disease and the use of steroids. Hyperglycemia causes excessive thirst, excessive urination and excessive hunger. Hypoglycemia (low blood sugar) can be caused by too much insulin, poor diet, and underactive thyroid. Symptoms of hypoglycemia include slurred speech, weakness, decreased level of consciousness, fainting, nervousness, and sweating.

Hemoglobin and erythrocytes

Hemoglobin should normally range between 13.5-18.0 for men and 12.0 - 16.0 for women. Decreased levels of Hgb and Hct. indicate anemia, or blood loss, reducing the oxygen carrying capacity of the blood. Severely anemic patients or those with excessive blood loss require oxygen. Too many erythrocytes or RBC's cause the blood to become thicker, producing an increased workload (afterload) of the heart. Abnormally high red blood cell count is referred to as polycythemia, and is seen in patients with COPD and with some congenital heart disease. Thickened blood makes your patient more prone to dangerous clots that could potentially enter the pulmonary system or cause ischemia to vital organs. Normal RBC count is 4.2 -5.2 for women and 4.6 - 6.2 for men.

Abnormal clotting blood tests

Before you draw blood or perform any procedures that could cause bruising or bleeding, check the patient's coagulation studies. Values: APTT (activated partial thromboplastin time) = 30-40 secs, PTT (partial thromboplastin time) = 60 70 secs, Bleeding = 1-3 minutes. The PT = 11 -12.5 secs. Patients who are receiving Coumadin (Warfarin) blood thinner will receive frequent PT testing to keep the INR within a certain range for prevention of clot formation. The respiratory therapist needs to monitor these values closely and consider the patient's condition when providing testing and treatment. Precautions must be taken to prevent bleeding. Elevations in the WBC (white blood cells) indicate infection. WBC's are also called leukocytes. Severe infection is present when the WBC count is >17,000 in adults. A low WBC count is often the result of a virus. It can be indicative of low immunity. Low WBC's in the blood makes the patient more vulnerable to infection, so take extra care using aseptic technique. Normal WBC count is 4,500 – 11,000 for adults and 9,000 – 33,000 in infants.

Laboratory culture and gram stain

The respiratory therapist may be responsible for obtaining a sputum specimen to test for bacterial lung infection. Gram stain provides rapid identification of aggressive infections. When the culture is complete, the results will be returned along with a list of antibiotics that can be used to effectively treat the infection (culture and sensitivity testing). This is especially important if pneumonia or bronchitis is present. Other fluids that may require a gram stain, culture and sensitivity include pleural fluid and blood. Most pneumonias and bronchitis are caused by Gram positive (Gm+) bacteria, treated with antibiotics. In the laboratory, the fluid or sputum is placed on a slide and the bacteria are "stained". Gram+ bacteria result in a purple stain. Gram negative (Gm-) bacteria are more aggressive, because they are opportunistic and are found in patients who are weak or chronically and severely ill. They require specific antibiotics that cover a wider range of bacteria; in other words a broad spectrum antibiotic. Culture results take 48 hours. Special testing is needed for tuberculosis, aspergillus and fungal diseases. The results take several weeks.

Pulmonary function results

Pulmonary function testing

Patients who are diagnosed with lung disease have at least a twenty percent variance from the predicted normal lung measurements. Specifically, those with obstructive lung disease will have pulmonary testing results (FRC, RV, and TLC) higher than the predicted values. Conversely, smaller values are seen in the presence of restrictive lung disease.

The patient with asthma will have a decrease in vital capacity and expiratory reserve volume. The patient with COPD will show increased FRC and RV. Functional residual capacity is increased because of air trapping. The ratio of RV to TLC is a better determinant of the diagnosis of specific types of disease because of the relationship between the two volumes. Consideration of each value alone may be misleading when the TLC is proportionately increased or decreased. Remember that normal RV total ratio is 20%:35%.

Pulmonary function changes

Reserve volume to total lung capacity is increased (RV:TLC) with asthma. Vital capacity (VC) is diminished. The inspiratory capacity is normal. Functional residual capacity may be normal or increased. Expiratory reserve capacity (ERV) is decreased. With COPD, results vary depending on how advanced the disease is. All pulmonary function is decreased in severe cases of COPD. Early changes show decreased FRC. Obesity causes a decrease in ERV. FRC may be increased or normal. Thus RV:TLC capacity is increased. Nitrogen washout distribution testing (sbN2) allows a more accurate measurement of the severity of emphysema or other restrictive lung disease by providing more information about the health of the small airways. A nitrogen analyzer is used to measure how much nitrogen is exhaled after inspiratory vital capacity of 100% O2.

Alveolar-arterial oxygen partial pressure difference

The alveolar-arterial pressure difference is the gradient between alveolar oxygenation and arterial oxygenation. [P (A-a) O2] This measurement defines the efficiency of the lungs and defines the seriousness of your patient's respiratory condition. When the patient who is receiving high levels of oxygen develops refractory hypoxemia you will see an increase in the partial pressure difference. This is a key to determining if the patient should be intubated.

To determine the partial pressure gradient, use the following method: Identify the PO2 and PCO2 on blood gas analysis. Note the patient's body temperature. Use a reference table when the temperature is not normal, otherwise 47mmHg (torr) is used in your analysis. Check the percent of inspired oxygen and use 0.8 as the value for the respiratory exchange ratio; this is the amount a normal person uses. You should calculate exchange ratio whenever possible, or if you're asked to do so. This determines the water vapor pressure (Ph2). Measure the Pb (local barometric pressure in mmHg. (torr). Obtain the patient's PAO2 using the following equation:

$$(PAO2 = [Pb - Ph2) \times FIO2] - \frac{PCO2}{.8}$$

Now subtract the PaO2 from the PA02 to obtain your result.

The partial pressure difference should be no more than 15 torr in a normal young person. Lung disease causes significant increases and some increase is normal with aging. Lung conditions that cause increased oxygen/alveolar pressure gradient include ARDS and ventricular septal defects The following will reveal a low ventilation to perfusion ratio on room air, causing an elevated P(A-a)O2: Pulmonary fibrosis, asthma, bronchitis, emphysema. Hypoxic patients who are hypoventilated have a normal P(A-a)O2 on room air. Providing oxygen supplementation corrects the low PaO2. You should suspect ARDS or other anatomical shunt if oxygen administration does not correct an elevated P(A-a)O2. A gradient of more than 350 torr indicates the presence of refractory hypoxemia. If high levels of oxygen are already being provided (80-100%), consider mechanical ventilatory support. Remember, increased A-a gradient means pulmonary disease; true shunting, resulting in ventilation/perfusion mismatch >30% is not responsive to increased oxygen delivery. Positive pressure to maximize lung volume is needed.

MEP

MEP is the "maximum expiratory pressure", the total amount of pressure a person can exert with forceful exhalation. It measures muscular strength and helps determine whether a patient can be weaned from the ventilator. Your patient must be willing and able to provide effort; muscle strength must be adequate and ventilatory drive must be present. Use a double one way valve with a manometer for a ventilated patient in order to allow inhalation while blocking exhalation. Explain the procedure. Use a gauge that measures at least 60cm. of water pressure. Instruct your patient to breath around the mouthpiece and provide a nose clip. The patient must seal the device with his teeth and lips. The patient inhales completely and breathes out with as much force as possible, holding for 1 to 3 seconds. Get three good efforts. Document the most stable value measured after one second of effort and observe vital signs. Normal MEP should produce at least + 80cm. of water pressure, regardless of age or gender; +40cm is acceptable.

Preductal and postductal oxygenation studies

The PO2 is measured in the preductal and postductal blood. Measurements of preductal blood are obtained from the right radial artery, right arm or right upper chest probe or pulse oximeter on the right hand. Postductal blood is done by sampling the umbilical artery, or applying a pulse oximeter to the feet or left hand. A probe can be placed on the thighs or abdomen. PPHN is determined by a 10% decrease in SPO2 from pre to postductal blood, or a greater than 15 to 20 torr decrease from pre to post ductal blood. The test is not definitive. Abnormal results indicate a need for further testing.

Incentive spirometry

Incentive spirometry allows your patient to expand the lungs. The patient can visually see results on the device. Evidence shows that incentive spirometry is best used to treat existing atelectasis. Effective instruction must be provided to your patient. Set a goal that your patient can easily reach, but one that requires at least moderate effort. Have the patient breathe in deeply and slowly. Demonstrate proper breathing using the correct muscles. At this point, you can demonstrate which accessory muscles should be avoided. Once maximal inspiration is attained, have the patient hold it for 5-10 seconds then exhale normally. Let your patient rest before the next exercise. The frequency needed for each patient may vary, but a general rule is 5-10 exercises per hour. Observe your patient's progress periodically and document your findings. Make certain the spirometer is always within patient reach and note vital signs during the procedure. Document your patient's vital signs during supervised sessions. Minimal supervision should be required following the initial instruction.

The most obvious reason to stop incentive spirometry is that the patient no longer needs it and has met goals. Some patients may need to continue at home. If the patient becomes short of breath or develops chest pain, assess breath sounds. Be aware that pneumothorax could develop. If the patient develops numbness or tingling from rapid breathing, the therapist should discontinue spirometry. Other reasons may become evident, such as extreme weakness, inability to remove the oxygen source because O2 saturation drops and intolerance from pain. The last can be avoided by timing the treatment with the healthcare team. Schedule a treatment after the patient has received a mild pain medication. It is important for the patient to be alert during treatment. Anytime the treatment does not benefit the patient, make a recommendation for an alternative therapy to treat atelectasis.

FVC and VC tests

FVC (Forced Vital Capacity) is the amount of air exhaled rapidly after a full inhalation. VC (Vital Capacity Pulmonary Function Test) is the measurement of exhaled gas after maximum inhalation. It is done slowly. The test is performed either with a regular spirometer or with a computerized spirometer that provides printed test results. Under normal circumstances, the two results should be the same. FVC declines with age. Diminished FVC is seen in patients with COPD, asthma, cystic fibrosis and bronchiectasis. Determine the predicted value of FVC in a patient and compare it to the actual results by dividing the result by the predicted test value, then multiply x 100. When the result is over 80%, it is within normal range. Predicted FVC values are adjusted and measured automatically when patient information is entered into the pulmonary function testing device. When you look at the FVC tracing, it should show a line going straight up at the start of exhalation. When restrictive or obstructive disease is present, exhalation is slow and it is reflected by a more horizontal tracing.

FEV1

FEV1 is the measurement of the amount of gas the patient is able to exhale within one second of inhalation of total lung capacity. It is reported after three good attempts are provided by the patient. The highest value is recorded. FEV1 is the most frequently used pulmonary function test to determine bronchoconstriction (COPD), bronchodilatation, or to assess airway obstruction. It is performed using forced exhalation. FEV1, along with FVC measurement is used as a test to determine how well the patient has responded to bronchodilators. When improvement of 15% or more is seen, reversible airway obstruction is present.

Diagnosis of pulmonary disease includes a combination of measurements, including peak flow, (PF), forced expiratory volume (FEVT), forced expiratory flow (FEF), and forced expiratory volume, forced vital capacity ratio (FEVT/FVC): combined with the clinical picture, evaluation of radiographs, and blood gas analysis. Remember that obstructive disease shows increases >120% in RV, FRC and TLC. Restrictive lung disease results in FRC, RV and TLC at <80% of the patient's predicted value.

I:E ratio

The I:E ratio is the difference between the amount of time a patient breathes in and breathes out. It is measured while the patient uses a spirometer while the respiratory therapist uses a watch to time the breathing cycle. It takes a longer time to breathe in when upper airway obstruction is present. Expiratory times are increased with COPD and asthma. A diabetic with Kussmaul breathing is an example of a patient you would expect to have an abnormal I:E ratio. Normally, the I:E ratio range is between 1:2 and 1:4. If it takes 2 seconds to breathe in and 10 seconds to breathe out, the I:E ratio would be 1:5. If a patient's I:E ratio is abnormal, the cause should be investigated.

DLCO

A test that measures the diffusing capacity of the blood (DLCO), allows the physician to obtain more information about the severity of pulmonary disease. Blood acts as a barrier to the diffusion of oxygen. Carbon monoxide (CO) binds to hemoglobin, providing a better means to observe the rate at which the gas passes through the pulmonary capillaries. The results are then compared to determine the rate that oxygen passes through the lungs. Conditions such as emphysema, pulmonary fibrosis, anemia, and pulmonary hypertension will result in a reduction of DLCO. The test is easy for the patient to perform because it requires a single breath, when compared to spirometry which requires more effort. The patient performs the test in an upright position. A single breath of a small amount carbon monoxide is inhaled while the breath is held for ten seconds. Upon exhalation, the expired gases are separated by the gas sampler to acquire the DLCO reading. RV and TLC are measured prior to the test.

Pulmonary artery pressure

The pulmonary artery pressure catheter provides measurement of CVP, left ventricular diastolic pressure, cardiac output and the individual components that define cardiac output - stroke volume and cardiac index (the amount of blood ejected from the left ventricle in one minute). The proximal port of the CVP catheter lies in the right atrium. The distal port lies in the pulmonary artery and measures systolic, diastolic and pulmonary capillary wedge pressure. The CVP port is used to administer I.V. medications and fluid. A connector is attached to the pulmonary artery catheter and to a computer to measure cardiac output (CO). PVR (pulmonary vascular resistance) is calculated by the difference between pulmonary artery diastolic pressure and the PCWP. The balloon port is used to measure PCWP. It can be used to draw blood for mixed venous sampling. The tubing must be properly assembled and maintained. A transducer, placed at mid chest level provides consistent and accurate readings. When the equipment is moved, or the patient is repositioned the transducer must be again leveled at midchest to provide correct readings.

An improperly placed transducer, or tubing that contains air, will render pulmonary pressure readings abnormal. If the transducer is below the mid chest mark the reading will be falsely high. Increased pulmonary artery pressure is the result of congestive heart failure, volume overload, and decreased cardiac output. Decreased pulmonary artery pressure can be the result of shock and is accompanied by low blood pressure.

PCWP readings are taken by inflating the balloon at the tip of the catheter with the recommended amount of air. This blocks the blood flow in the pulmonary artery and should be done as quickly as possible to prevent ischemia and injury to the pulmonary segment. Results that are elevated are indicative of volume overload, congestive heart failure and insufficiency of the mitral valve.

Decreased PCWP occurs from hypovolemia or sepsis (low cardiac output state).

Plethysmography

Plethysmography is used to measure lung volumes. The patient is asked to breathe inside an airtight chamber. The then measures volume difference within the chamber. The unit must be airtight to obtain accurate measurements of TGV and RAW. The calculations are performed by obtaining TGV, then calculating FRV and TV from the result. The patient breathes into a pneumotachometer to obtain FRC and the system then closes to prevent air leaks after exhalation. After the system closes, the patients breathing efforts are continued while the pressures in the plethysmograph are calculated. TGV results are greater than FRC if gas trapping is present. The unit must be calibrated to provide accurate results. The patient must be properly instructed so that the test is properly performed. When these criteria are met, plethysmography provides an accurate measurement of FRC. A computer is used to assimilate the data.

When performing body plethysmography, the patient is asked breathe after swallowing a balloon connected, to a catheter. The balloon is injected with air. It is connected to a transducer. During breathing, the transducer measures changes in the patient's intrathoracic pressure. Once the patient is placed in the plethysmograph unit the lung volume is measured by the pneumotachometer. As the patient inhales and then exhales, the pneumotachometer system is intermittently open and closed to measure pressure inside the chest as lung volume increases and decreases. Lung and thoracic compliance (CL and CT) in a normal adult =.2L/cm H2O. Since the chest expands with breathing, and the lungs become smaller, the equation lung/thoracic compliance becomes 0.1L/cmH2O to offset the difference. The patient's history and physical, combined with the results of lung compliance and other pulmonary function tests provide a definitive diagnosis of lung function.

Aneroid pressure manometer

The aneroid manometer is used to measure lung pressures. Lung measurements are obtained by calibrating the manometer which is spring loaded, and attaching it to a pressure source. The results are displayed in either mmHg or cm H2O. When connecting a manometer to a pressure source it must be airtight to display an accurate reading. Manometers can be checked for accuracy by attaching the gauge to a mercury sphygmomanometer and matching the gauge and the sphygmomanometer for duplicate readings. You can also open the manometer and "zero" it to room air. If a manometer gauge can't be calibrated it should not be used. When proper calibration fails, recheck all of the connections. The presence of air leaks when using any pulmonary function equipment will provide inaccurate readings.

Water seal spirometer

Water seal spirometers provide a printed graph of the patient's breathing. New units automatically calculate the results. Specialty gases can be added to the units to test residual volume and diffusion capacities. The units contain a removable filter to absorb CO2. If the test is performed for less than fifteen seconds the filter will not be needed, but otherwise must be in place to prevent the patient from breathing CO2 and becoming short of breath. If FVC testing is performed, remove the CO2 filter to allow the free flow of gas. As with all equipment, make sure all connections are secure. The water level in the unit must be precise for accuracy.

Nitrogen washout test

The first phase of the test is used to measure vital capacity. The patient exhales oxygen from the dead space after breathing 100% oxygen. Once pure oxygen is exhaled nitrogen follows from the alveoli, mixing with the dead space. The first 750 ml. of gas are not used in the measurements. Once the gases are stabilized in the lungs, the third phase of the test is performed by measuring the increase in nitrogen found in 500 ml. of gas. The amount of Nitrogen is increased with advanced lung disease. Results of 6-10% are usually indicative of emphysema. The nitrogen is measured further during this phase once 30% of VC is exhaled. Phase four is considered the end of respiratory effort. During this time nitrogen levels greatly increase until the residual volume is depleted providing closure of the airways. This is the closing volume. The airways should not close before 80 to 90% of gas is exhaled. The patient's history and clinical presentation is considered in conjunction with the test results to obtain a definite diagnosis.

Blood gas results

Blood gas analysis provides much information. Any injury or illness that affects oxygenation or metabolic status is an indication for blood gas analysis. When obtaining a blood gas, arterial blood is used. Capillary blood that is oxygenated can be used for analysis in newborns. When drawing blood for analysis make certain the sample is correctly drawn from the artery and not the vein. Information obtained from blood gas includes metabolic status, respiratory status and level of oxygenation. To withdraw blood from a central or radial catheter, sterile techniques must be used. Infection is a risk if septic technique is not used at all times. Remember to waste the first 5ml.of blood withdrawn from the catheter, and then obtain your sample. Air in the syringe will provide an incorrect blood gas result.

The specimen must be tested within ten minutes, otherwise place it on ice to prevent the consumption of oxygen in the sample. Use aseptic technique and universal precautions for infection control.

Arterial puncture

When using arterial puncture for ABG sampling, use aseptic technique and sterile equipment. Prepare the site with alcohol and iodine. Use gloves and protective eye wear to prevent the possibility of eye, mouth or nose contamination. Make sure all the equipment is within reach, including a cup of ice. Blood is usually sampled from the radial artery. Perform the Allen's test and document the results. Blood thinners are widely used in the hospital and at home. It's important to know the patient's coagulation status. Improper technique can result in patient infection or accidental needle puncture. Use universal precautions. Advance the needle carefully. Cap the syringe immediately after the blood is drawn. Aggressive needle insertion can damage the artery. Apply direct pressure to the site for 3-5 minutes or longer when needed. Dispose of all biohazardous material. Arterial spasm is painful to the patient and should be noted. Blood clots in the artery can also develop. Look for signs of hematoma and document any complications.

Infant considerations

Infants with pulmonary disease require blood gas analysis, but the size of their small arteries makes direct sampling impossible. Blood can be obtained by lancing the earlobe, heel, finger or the great toe. These are considered areas with good blood supply or vascularization and are used to sample arterialized capillary blood. Samples are obtained by using a pediatric lance. The area should be warmed before the sample is taken. A heat lamp or warm towel should suffice. Use aseptic technique then lance the area. Use a capillary tube and let the blood flow freely into the tube so you don't express venous blood during the collection. Obtain two tubes. Seal the tubes then mix the blood. Apply pressure for bleeding. Place the capillary tubes on ice. If you are using the foot, avoid the middle of the foot. This is where the posterior tibial artery is located. Send the sample to the laboratory for testing.

Reanalyzing results

You may be asked to reanalyze blood gas results that don't fit a patient's clinical presentation or are otherwise questionable. Consider the following to ensure results are always accurate. Two different analyzers can be used for comparison. Check the blood gas analyzer carefully to make sure that all quality controls have been consistently met. Records are kept each time controls are performed. Adhere to the steps outlined by the manufacturer and make sure they are followed to prevent errors. If one point calibration is not automatic, it should be performed before every test. Two point calibration should generally be performed every eight hours or after 25 samples have been tested. Three point calibration is mandated every six months or when new electrodes are used. Review the equipment for proper function and repeat the test.

Carbon monoxide poisoning

Carbon monoxide poisoning requires a different approach to blood gas analysis. It is treated and diagnosed very specifically. Carbon monoxide adheres to hemoglobin in the red blood cells, just as oxygen does. The result is a state of carboxyhemoglobinemia. If carbon monoxide poisoning is suspected, the pulse oximeter will display a false reading. A patient who has inhaled carbon monoxide will show falsely adequate oxygenation as displayed on the pulse ox. It is necessary to perform a blood gas analysis using a CO oximeter. The CO oximeter allows accurate measurement of the hemoglobin characteristics and can be used to diagnose hemoglobin abnormalities, such as methemoglobin. To obtain an accurate reading with the CO oximeter, follow the instructions given by the manufacturer.

Imaging studies

Chest x-ray (radiograph)

A respiratory therapist would recommend a chest x-ray if tension pneumothorax is suspected. Tension pneumothorax can result from inhaled foreign object, trauma, and tumor blocking the airway, and swelling of the larynx, spontaneously or following cardiopulmonary procedures. The air in the pleura becomes rapidly greater than the atmospheric pressure, causing a shift in the trachea and mediastinum. The resultant shift can compress the heart and blood vessels and lead to death. Mechanical ventilation with positive pressure can cause a tension pneumothorax as well. The symptoms of pneumothorax include tracheal deviation, or a shift from the normal midline position. The patient may have chest pain and will be short of breath. Upon exam, breath sounds will be absent. The chest may move in a paradoxical fashion or asymmetrically. When you palpate the chest, you will feel increased resonance over the affected lung field. Look for a sudden rise in peak pressures. Recommend a chest x-ray to confirm endotracheal tube placement, following the placement of a chest tube, worsening patient condition, bloody sputum (hemoptysis) and insertion of a pulmonary artery catheter.

Radiograph views

If a chest x-ray is underexposed, the body tissues will appear too white Overexposure makes the tissues and lung fields appear black. On the lateral X-Ray, the patient's left side is against the film cassette and the arms are overhead to better view the heart. The lateral decubitus X-ray of the chest will reveal small amounts of fluid. The patient is positioned on either side or in the dorsal position for this view. A dorsal decubitus X-ray view is used to identify pneumothorax in infants. The lordotic view of the chest is used to see the upper lungs. This view excludes structures that may obscure the upper lungs. It provides a view of the lung apices. The patient is tilted slightly back and the X-Ray is directed upward. Oblique views of the chest are performed with the patient rotated to the right or left.

Oblique views are ordered when the edges of the heart and mediastinal structures require scrutiny and when looking tumors, cysts or other lung masses.

Chest x-ray findings

Look at the position of the endotracheal tube. The endotracheal tube should be seen inside the tracheal lumen, halfway between the larynx and the bifurcation of the trachea. The chest x-ray results to the previous. Check for air in the pleura, mediastinum and in the soft tissues. Pneudomediastinum is air in the mediastinal space. Pneumopericardium is air in the pericardial sac. Air outside of the abdominal area or peritoneum is pneumoperitoneum. Air in the soft tissue can be the result of alveolar rupture from mechanical ventilation. It can also be the result of procedures that require needle insertion, such as pulmonary artery catheter insertion. Look for displacement of tubes (chest, feeding, pulmonary catheters). Check for the presence of new infiltrates, edema or pulmonary consolidation. Centrally placed I.V. catheters should be seen in their entirety on X-ray. Mediastinal shift is abnormal. Tracheal deviation occurs when the mediastinal structures shift from tension pneumothorax, atelectasis, or fluid. The mediastinum normally appears left of center in adults, and is centered in newborns.

Opinion of sample x-ray

The x-ray is taken with a lateral view. The radiograph shows a narrowing of the tracheal air column below the larynx. The upper airway is clear until the level of the trachea. You also can see that the air column appears sharp. The patient is a six year old who was admitted after a five day history of fever and cough. The patient has no previous medical history, and has been admitted with shortness of breath.

Suspect croup because of the appearance of narrowing and the "pencil sign" below the vocal cords. Croup or laryngotracheobronchitis causes swelling of the vocal cords. It is differentiated from epiglottitis because of the location of the swelling. Epiglottitis produces swelling above the vocal cords with a normal appearance in the tracheal air column. The upper airway appears hazy instead of clear when epiglottitis is present. Clinically, epiglottitis develops suddenly. X-Ray of the airway should show a normal, dark column. You should recommend that your patient be evaluated for left sided heart failure. Left heart enlargement is abnormal in a patient of this age. Other x-ray findings would be evident if there were effusions or infiltrates, such as haziness and shadowing.

EKGs

EKG electrodes

The EKG provides a tracing of the heart from all views. The only view that requires special electrode placement is the posterior view. Standard electrocardiograph tracings are performed as a baseline in older patients. Symptoms that could indicate an M.I. include dyspnea, diaphoresis, left arm or jaw pain, abdominal pain, syncope, and even upper or low back pain. There are four limb leads and six precordial, or chest leads. Reversing the limb leads will display false information. Interference from patient movement should be minimized during the test. If electrical interference is seen, check for proper grounding. The patient's skin must be dry and free of oil to obtain diagnostic EKG tracings.

Normal EKG characteristics

The normal EKG consists of a P wave, QRS complex, ST segment, then T wave. Normal resting heart rate is between 60 and 100bpm. The QRS complexes are upright in Lead II of the EKG. The distance between QRS complexes should be regular. It's normal to have a slight irregularity (sinus arrhythmia) with breathing, especially in younger persons. The QRS complexes should be narrow, and they should look the same. When the rate is above 100, the EKG appears normal; only the rate increases. Hypoxia, hypotension, pain, and fever can all increase the heart rate, causing sinus tachycardia. Sinus bradycardia on EKG would also appear normal, but the rate falls below 60 bpm. In the absence of symptoms, no treatment is necessary. It's important to know your patient's baseline heart rate. Vagal stimulation frequently occurs during suctioning and coughing. Critically ill patients should be observed for episodes of bradycardia related vagal (parasympathetic) stimulation.

Monitoring data

Pulmonary mechanics

<u>Lung compliance</u>

Lung compliance is diminished in patients with asthma, COPD, ARDS, pulmonary fibrosis, pneumonia and pulmonary edema. Lung compliance values include static compliance (normal adult 100ml.cm.H20). Infant CLT is normally 5ml/cmH20. Static compliance is the combination of CLT and thoracic compliance. Dynamic compliance is the result of airway resistance and static compliance. Measurement of lung compliance tells the respiratory therapist how easily tidal volumes can be delivered and assists in measuring improvement or worsening patient condition. Find the compliance factor by first measuring the tidal volume then dividing it by peak pressure. Remember that peak pressure includes subtracting any PEEP and takes into account lost volume from ventilator circuitry (compressed volume). Once lung compliance is determined measure dynamic compliance:

$$Cdyn = \text{exhaled VT – compressed volume (previously calculated)}$$
$$\text{Plateau pressure – PEEP}$$

<u>MVV</u>

MVV is maximum voluntary ventilation. It is a pulmonary function test used to determine how much gas is exhaled in a specified amount of time, usually fifteen seconds. The minimum amount of time is five seconds. Multiply the result to determine the volume exhaled in one minute, i.e. 15 x 4 or 5 x 12. The results are often non specific because of variables in the patient's effort during the test. MVV results that are less than 70% of predicted are considered abnormal, but are not very specific in providing a diagnosis. MVV can be useful to determine if a patient can undergo stress testing and to assess for pre-operative pulmonary risk. The patient who is weak or has neuromuscular disease will not be able to reach vital capacity easily. The results may be lower due to fatigue. A true effort from the patient is needed and the respiratory therapist must render an opinion of good effort.

Respiratory monitoring

Vd/Vt ratio

The Vd/Vt ratio is the ratio of dead space to tidal volume. Several conditions cause variances in the expected percentage of dead space. The amount of dead space can be a factor in deciding whether to provide mechanical ventilation to a patient. Normal adults have a ratio of dead space to tidal volume of 20 to 40% while newborn's have 30%. Calculation of 60% or greater of dead space is a predictor of impending respiratory failure. A volumetric capnometer provides computerized calculation of the dead space. Record the results and draw a blood gas for analysis. Conditions that increase the amount of dead space include pulmonary embolism and tumors. The dead space increases quickly when pulmonary embolism develops. Less dead space becomes available when there is bronchoconstriction (asthma), lung resection or pneumonectomy, or when a tracheal tube or endotracheal tube is in place.

Mechanical dead space

Mechanical dead space is added when ABG results show that the patient is being overly ventilated and the CO2 level falls. This is accomplished by adding tubing to the ventilator circuitry and increasing the oxygen flow to compensate for the increased amount of exhaled CO2. Adding mechanical dead space is done only during control and assist control ventilator modes. To calculate the amount of dead space needed, plug the patient data into the following formula:

$$(VT - VD[anatomic]) \text{ -- } (VD[mechanical]) \text{ x f x } PaCO2 =$$
$$(VT - VD[anatomic]) - (VD[\text{desired mechanical dead space}]) \text{ x f x desired } PaCO2$$

Note that in the first equation actual values are used. The patient's anatomic dead space should be calculated as 2.2ml/kg. body weight. In the second part of the equation, desired values are used. The result will tell you how many ml. of dead space should be added to obtain the desired PaCO2 level.

Increased or decreased physiological dead space

Calculation of Vd/Vt provides a measurement of wasted ventilation. Mechanical ventilation is indicated if the Vd/Vt ratio is 60% or greater. Total dead space is the sum of the anatomical dead space and the alveolar dead space. This is known as physiological dead space. Typically, the patient's minute volume is increased but alveolar ventilation does not occur due to the absence of capillary blood flow in the alveoli or if airway narrowing is present. Breathing is shallow when the patient's minute volume increases. Mechanical ventilation decreases the Vd/Vt ratio because of the presence of the endotracheal tube, as does a tracheostomy tube. Normal anatomical dead space is approximately 150ml. A common cause of increased dead space is pulmonary embolism and the presence of tumors. Calculate by measuring the end tidal CO2 and PaCO2.
Use the equation:

$$Vd/Vt = PaCO2 - PetCO2 / PaCO2.$$

Noninvasive monitoring

Arterial end tidal CO2 gradient

Determination of the patient's arterial end tidal carbon dioxide gradient will help decide when to safely wean from mechanical ventilation. A patient who is hypoventilating after surgery will have an end tidal CO2 greater than the arterial CO2 because of incomplete exhalation. Obtain two blood gas samples: one to measure PaCO2 and one to measure PetCO2 – calculate the difference to obtain the gradient. Normal gradient is 1-5 torr or less. Determine the patient's baseline for comparison. Make sure the patient is stimulated to encourage deep breathing. When the end tidal CO2 gradient has been assessed, capnography can be used to monitor the patient's progress. Once the capnography system is placed for sampling, be certain to monitor the tracings for elevations in CO2. This will determine interventions and treatments necessary. Review how to analyze the results. Know the significance of abnormal waveforms that reflect changes in alveolar ventilation. Troubleshoot the equipment frequently by clearing the capillary tube of water or secretions; maintain airtight connections, and check for proper calibration.

Alveolar ventilation and minute volume

Changes in respiratory rate and tidal volume cause changes in alveolar ventilation, and alter CO2 levels in the blood. Va (Alveolar ventilation) refers to the tidal volume that travels to the alveoli. To determine Va, the patient's exhaled volume is measured and the amount of dead space is subtracted from the exhaled volume. Dead space is estimated to be 2.2ml/kg of healthy body weight, so a patient who weighs 90 kg. has a dead space of 198 ml. When the exhaled volume is 500 ml. the alveolar ventilation result is 302 ml.

VE (Minute volume) is the amount of volume of gas moving out of the lungs in one minute. It is measured using a spirometer and can be determined by multiplying the respiratory rate by the tidal volume.

Bedside cardiopulmonary monitoring

Bedside monitoring of a patient's cardiopulmonary status can be accomplished by insertion of a CVP (central venous pressure) catheter or by using a PA (pulmonary artery) catheter. The CVP catheter measures pressure in the right atrium and is valuable when medication and fluids must be rapidly administered. It is inserted into the right subclavian vein or into the right jugular vein. The pulmonary artery catheter is a balloon tipped catheter that measures pressures in the heart, and reflect the patient's cardiac and pulmonary status. It is called a Swan Ganz catheter. Patients who are mechanically ventilated and on multiple medications require close monitoring at the bedside to measure response to various therapies and during the post operative period.

Central venous pressure is measured in cm. H20 or mm/Hg. Normal CVP for infants is 1-5 mm/Hg, newborns 0-3, and adults 2-8. Normal pulmonary artery pressure is 15-28/5-17 mm/Hg. for adults, children 15-30/5-10 and newborns 30-60/2-10. The PAP measurement is the systolic and diastolic pressure in the pulmonary arteries. The distal catheter lies in the pulmonary artery when properly positioned.

Pulmonary capillary wedge pressure is obtained by inflating the balloon at the end of the catheter to briefly prevent blood flow to the ventricle. The normal value is 6-15mm/Hg. It is also referred to a pulmonary wedge pressure (PWP), pulmonary artery wedge pressure, (PAWP), pulmonary capillary wedge pressure (PCWP). When obtaining wedge pressures, it is imperative to remember to deflate the balloon entirely to prevent pulmonary infarct.

Capnography

Capnography is used to monitor Petco2. Attach an infrared sensor to the artificial airway Insert the sensor into the nostril to monitor patients who are not intubated. Petco2 is measured during exhalation and is displayed as waveforms on a graph. The waveforms are monitored for changes to determine patient status. Capnography is best utilized in the absence of ventilation perfusion mismatches. The arterial end tidal CO2 gradient must first be determined before relying on capnography. This provides a baseline and helps determine the accuracy during capnography. The Petco2 and arterial CO2 measurements are calculated simultaneously to determine the appropriateness of capnography. Look for dampening of the waveforms on the computerized graph. When waveforms don't return to baseline, check for blockage in the capillary tube. Obstruction that prevents gas from reaching the CO2 analyzer will result in an abnormal graph, such as during CPR and with bronchoconstrictive lung disease. Changes in end tidal CO2 volume require investigation is indicative of a change in alveolar ventilation.

Holter monitoring

A Holter monitor can be used when a patient experiences non emergent cardiac symptoms. A patient who has been experiencing shortness of breath, chest pain, syncope, palpitations or other non acute cardiac symptoms may benefit from outpatient evaluation before more costly or invasive testing is considered. Several types of monitors are available, including 24, 48 and 30 day event monitors. Event monitors can transmit tracings during symptoms or when the monitor alarms are triggered automatically. Holter monitors record either 24 or 48 hr continuous recording of the heart rate and rhythm during activity. Event monitor tracings are transmitted over the phone after the patient's EKG tracing is stored in the monitor. Proper instruction and secure electrode placement is needed for the monitor to properly record. The skin must be prepared by removing oils and taping electrodes to the patient's chest. Holter monitor kits are prepackaged and come with instructions regarding electrode placement. The patient should be told to keep a diary of any symptoms to compare to the time of EKG tracing.

Maternal and perinatal/neonatal data

Important terms

Perinatal is the time "around" the end of pregnancy. The last five months of pregnancy and the four weeks following delivery are considered to be the perinatal period. Primigravida is the term used for a woman's first pregnancy. It does not mean that the woman has experienced the birth of a full term infant. Primipara refers to the first delivery of the infant. Gravida refers to pregnancy. Para refers the actual delivery. Assessment of the mother during the antenatal period (pre-delivery) is an important indicator of the risk for complications during delivery and of the newborn's risks for respiratory complications.

Apgar scores

The Apgar scoring system is a scale of 0-7 and reflects heart rate, breathing effort, reflex response, strength of muscle, and color immediately after birth. Oxygen is measured in the newborn to ensure closure of the ductus arteriosus. The ductus arteriosus closes shortly after birth, equalizing arterial oxygenation throughout the body. In a newborn with PPHN (persistent pulmonary hypertension) the ductus arteriosus will not close completely.

Respiratory distress in a newborn

The Apgar score at five minutes reveals how the neonate's cardiopulmonary system is adjusting. After five minutes, a low score is a predictor of one month mortality.

Pneumothorax can be spotted in a newborn by transillumination. Hold a flashlight to the chest in a darkened room. If there is free air in the lung the light makes a halo effect. Suspected epiglottitis is an emergency requiring intubation. On x-ray a white haziness is seen above the glottis from the swelling (thumb sign). If the doctor suspects epiglottitis, the infant should remain in an upright position. If croup or laryngotracheal bronchitis is suspected a mist tent with cool aerosol and racemic epinephrine is the anticipated treatment. Suspect aspiration for any sudden onset of respiratory distress. Cough and stridor are evidence of aspiration. Lateral neck radiograph can help determine the presence of a foreign body. Metallic objects appear white and solid. Plastic, food and tumors will display an irregular appearing airway.

Mothers who are not healthy may not have healthy babies. Very young mothers and those over age 40 are more at risk for preterm delivery. Fetal monitoring provides assessment of complications to the newborn. Changes in fetal heart rate can signal problems. A rate > 160 may signal a heart defect; < 120, hypoxia or asphyxiation. Trauma is possible during delivery. A sample of amniotic fluid can be obtained to test for pulmonary status of the fetus. The fluid is analyzed for the presence of surfactant to see if alveolar cells are developed. Without surfactant, the newborn is prone to RDS. A low Apgar score is an indication that a newborn could develop respiratory distress. Review the Apgar score, amniocentesis, if available, maternal history, birth weight and results of fetal monitoring to anticipate respiratory distress in the newborn. Be prepared to recommend administration of surfactant to a newborn that develops symptoms of RDS. Examples of surfactants include Exosurf, Curosurf, Infasurf and Survanta and can be instilled directly through an endotracheal tube.

Neonate risks during premature labor

The mother who goes into labor before 38 weeks gestation is considered to be in premature labor. Delivery before term has a negative impact on the neonate. The mother will have a fetal heart rate monitor applied during labor by way of an electrode place on the abdomen. The FHR should vary with contractions, and fetal movement. Normal heart rate in utero is between 120 and 160 bpm. When contractions occur, the fetal heart rate slows down. Once the contraction ends, the fetal heart rate should to return to normal. When the heart rate takes longer to accelerate following a contraction, low Apgar scores and respiratory distress should be anticipated. The mother should be supported with oxygen and close observation of maternal vital signs is needed in addition to close fetal monitoring. The respiratory therapist should be prepared to provide respiratory support and close assessment of the neonate who is delivered prematurely. Be prepared to deliver CPR or deliver other forms of resuscitation.

Meconium aspiration

Meconium aspiration is seen in the newborn following fetal distress. The neonate can aspirate meconium from amniotic fluid during gasping. Post mature delivery can result in aspiration if the newborn passes meconium in the amniotic fluid. It may even occur as the result of the normal stress of delivery. As the neonate breathes in, the lungs expand, but exhalation is restricted as the bronchioles constrict and meconium blocks air from escaping. Airway resistance becomes increased, air becomes trapped and auto PEEP occurs. The lungs can become traumatized; air leaks can develop. Inspiratory flow rates must be reduced to prevent barotrauma. Expiratory times must be increased to prevent air trapping. Mechanical ventilation settings are determined by viewing the infant's chest x-ray and monitoring blood gases. The goal of ventilation is to keep the inspiratory flow and rate low wand the inspiratory and expiratory times should be prolonged. Frequent suctioning, pulmonary hygiene and ventilatory support are provided for several days until weaning is possible.

Transcutaneous monitoring

Transcutaneous monitoring of CO_2 and O_2 is frequently used to monitor newborns diagnosed with PDA. The ability to monitor changes in CO_2 and O_2 assists in the diagnosis of right to left shunt or coarctation of the aorta. Close monitoring of the newborn during changes in therapy are needed on a continuous basis and can be provided using this method. The adult patient can also be monitored transcutaneously for changes in oxygen status. Proper electrode placement is necessary for accurate results. To monitor an infant, the electrodes should be placed on the upper chest, abdomen or medial upper thigh where the tissue is well perfused. For preductal measurement of Ptco2, the right upper chest is used. Check the physicians' order. For adults, place the electrodes on the upper chest and medial aspect of the upper arm. As with pulse oximetry, avoid areas of poor perfusion. Inaccuracies result in the presence of low cardiac output or vasoconstriction. Proper electrode contact is necessary, so the skin must be clean and dry.

Equipment application and cleanliness

Selecting and Using Equipment

Assessing ventilator settings

A patient has just had surgery and is mechanically ventilated; you have assessed his ventilator settings, and the ABG results reveal the following:

Blood Gas	Vent settings
PH = 7.40	SIMV Mode
PCO2= 40	VT 850 ml
HCO3= 23	Rate 6
BE= -3	Total RR 18
PO2= 86	FIO2 40%
O2 sat= 96%	5cm PEEP

His weight is 85kg. (187lbs)

Leave everything as is. The PH is normal. If the CO2 level was low, you would need to adjust the tidal volume and/or respiratory rate. PEEP settings that are low, as in this instance are considered physiologic and prevent alveolar collapse.

Blood gas analyzers

PCO2 and O2 and blood gas analyzer calibration

Use a given PCO2 AND O2 value when performing the calibration of the blood gas analyzer. When performing the calibration use the following formulas:

PCO2 = (Pb [760 or adjust to your facility] – PH2O) x CO2%.

Ph2O varies with the patient's body temperature. When the patient's temperature is normal 98.6 degrees Fahrenheit, the water vapor pressure is 47 torr. To calibrate O2 use the same equation. Use a given oxygen percentage for the predicted O2 value. PO2 = (Pb [760 or adjust to your facility] – PH2O) x O2%. Perform calibrations according to the recommendations provided by the manufacturer of the equipment and document all results. Most calibration errors can be corrected by making sure there are no air bubbles in the system and by flushing with saline to make sure the membranes are clean.

Arterial catheters problems

Arterial catheters can be a portal for infection. The catheter can become loose and if it advances, can introduce bacteria into the blood stream. Aseptic technique is necessary to avoid problems with infection. If there are signs of infection, the catheter should be removed and the situation should be reported to the physician for appropriate antibiotic therapy. If connections are loose or pressure is not maintained on the IV bag containing heparin, blood will appear in the tubing. Check connections and make certain pressure is maintained above the tubing to prevent backflow. A loose connection could cause hemorrhage. Never flush the arterial catheter without first checking that blood can be withdrawn. It is possible for a clot to form and you can send it into the bloodstream if the catheter is occluded from a clot. If a clot is suspected, the catheter should be removed. Tubing and stopcocks should be changed every 24 to 48 hrs. to prevent sepsis. Never replace a stopcock that has become contaminated.

Respiratory therapy equipment

Equipment can be disinfected in the home with a 3:1 acetic acid (white vinegar) and water solution. Take the equipment apart first, then soak for one hour. Towel dry and expose the equipment to air. Hospital equipment that contacts skin can be wiped with an antimicrobial, such as isopropyl alcohol or Iodine. Pasteurization, hot water disinfection, is required by soaking for thirty minutes at 170 degrees F and can be used on equipment that isn't damaged by high temperatures. Cidex and Sonacide solution are brand names of glutaraldehyde products. They provide high level disinfection for equipment that cannot withstand high levels of heat, such as plastics. Sterilization of highly contaminated equipment is done by autoclave or by using sterilizing solutions. Sterilization is always needed when equipment has been in contact with a patient who has been diagnosed with a Bacillus or Clostridium bacterial infection. Plastic equipment cannot be sterilized in an autoclave. Sterilizing solutions are required and the equipment must be completely immersed. Follow the guidelines provided by the manufacturer for proper sterilization.

Medical gas humidifiers

Jet humidifiers and bubble humidifiers are used to counteract the dryness of medical gas. Sterile water is aerosolized to break it into small droplets. Bubble humidifiers are replaced when the water is evaporated. When using a nasal cannula always humidify if the patient expresses discomfort. If more than 4l/min oxygen is being delivered nasally or by mask, it should be humidified. Jet humidifiers supply more moisture than bubble humidifiers at higher flow rates. Underwater jet humidifiers provide the highest level of humidity. Infection can be easily spread by aerosol if the water and humidifier are not changed every day. A heater can supply warmer oxygen if needed. Patients with artificial airways must receive warm, humidified oxygen. Various devices are available to supply large volume humidity. When providing humidity, the tubing can become full of condensation and block oxygen delivery. Replace or clear the tubing as needed   Aerosolized equipment must be checked frequently to make sure water levels are adequate. Aerosol masks are available but the oxygen flow must be set higher. Delivered oxygen percentages should be analyzed when possible.

Inspired percentage of oxygen

Inspired oxygen can become diluted with room air. Analyzing the amount of gas will ensure that the proper FIO2 is being delivered. Samples of gas should be taken close to the patient for accuracy. Various types of analyzers are available. When using any gas analyzer, become familiar with the operation by reading the information supplied by the manufacturer. As with all respiratory equipment, insure accuracy by properly calibrating the equipment. Troubleshoot calibration errors by checking the capillary tube for patency when using electric or paramagnetic analyzers. The only analyzers that are safe to use in the operating room are paramagnetic analyzers. Because electrochemical analyzers have electric alarm systems they are not recommended for use around flammable gases. Familiarize yourself with the equipment used in your facility. It is not possible to measure the oxygen delivery when using a nasal cannula, mask, nonrebreather mask or a partial rebreather. When removing the oxygen supply, limit the amount of time the patient is without oxygen and watch for signs of oxygen desaturation.

Medical gas regulation problems

If you have a problem identifying the contents of any medical gas cylinder, check the label. Cylinders and bulk oxygen supplies piped through hospitals contain devices to control the amount of pressure, or backflow as a safety measure. Hospital systems have backup sources of oxygen in case of failure. In the hospital, an alarm will sound when piped oxygen delivery fails or if the pressure becomes too high. Both air and oxygen are piped through hospital systems. Make certain the proper outlet and equipment is ready for assembly when providing gas administration at the bedside. Turn off valves immediately if a leak becomes evident. When transporting a patient, obtain a flow meter that can be laid flat. The Bourdon flow meter should be used. Check the meter first for proper functioning. Other flow meters will display inaccurate readings if not in the upright position. Remember that is always the respiratory therapist's job to check proper operation of equipment to insure patient safety.

Gas cylinder flow

Gas cylinders can become depleted during patient transport. It is important to know how much time is available before the patient will need a new cylinder. Note the patient's flow rate, how many pounds per square inch of gas are contained in the cylinder (L/psig) and note the pressure on the gauge. You will use the same factors no matter what type of cylinder is being used. Simply multiply the gauge pressure (psig) x pounds per square inch (L/psig) and divide the result by the liter flow. A patient with 2 liters oxygen flow, using a cylinder with an L/psig. of 1.36 and a gauge pressure of 1200 psig would have 816 minutes of oxygen flow available, or 13.6 hours. The equation looks like this:

$$\frac{1.36 * 1200}{2L} = \frac{816}{60} = 13.6$$

Oxygen delivery devices

A simple oxygen mask fits on the face, covering the nose and mouth. Proper fit is important for comfort and accurate oxygen delivery. Humidity is used. Set the flow meter at 5-10L/min to obtain a range of 35-60% oxygen delivery. Because of this variance, it's important to check the patient's status with pulse oximetry and ABG analysis. Be prepared to recommend changes in the oxygen delivery device as patient condition changes. Side ports in the mask allow for the inhalation of room air and provide an outlet for exhaled air. Also, if the oxygen source becomes disconnected the patient still has access to room air.

The non rebreather mask can deliver up to 80% oxygen. Pure oxygen is delivered to the reservoir which is attached to the mask. There are no escape ports so the patient breathes pure oxygen in theory, but some room air is likely to enter unless the mask is fitted tightly. Humidity is also used with a non rebreather. The flow must be set high. If the reservoir collapses, increase the flow. Monitor the patient's oxygenation status.

Oxygen is delivered to a tracheostomy with the use of aerosolized T-piece or a tracheostomy collar. The T-piece delivers a mist around the tracheotomy site. It's important to check the equipment before applying. Aerosol should be visible. Carbon dioxide is inhaled if the nebulizer is not adequately filled with sterile water or if oxygen flow is not high enough. Remember to adjust the flow and check the air entrainment nebulizer if aerosol is not being delivered. The T-piece can also be used with an endotracheal tube. The tracheostomy collar is fitted over the trachea, is also aerosolized with an air entrainment nebulizer and should be adjusted the same way as the T-piece to ensure proper oxygenation. It's recommended that you check the oxygen percentage inside the mask to determine the needed flow.

The partial rebreathing mask is designed like the non rebreather, with the exception of the presence of side ports that contain either one, or two one-way valves. The valves prevent the patient from breathing room air, but provide a means for exhaled gas to escape. The reservoir is filled with oxygen, ready for delivery with each patient breath. There is a valve that will "pop off" if the oxygen supply is disconnected, allowing the patient to obtain room air. Set the flow meter high enough to fill the reservoir with oxygen, and then place it on the patient. Check for proper fit. Masks are available to accommodate pediatric and adult patients. Use a humidifier. When choosing a device for oxygen delivery, remember the goal is to maintain the PaO_2 between 50 and 60% (torr). If the patient is being monitored with oximetry, reassess immediately if the SpO_2 falls below 85%. Patients with COPD often are maintained with some level of hypoxemia, making them the exception. Report concerns to the physician and review your patient's history.

Air compressors and air/oxygen blenders

Air compressors can be used in the home to deliver nebulizers and IPPB therapy. They are used to deliver gas other than oxygen, and deliver room air that travels through a filter. High powered piston compressors are used in the hospital for the air that is piped into the hospital system. In the home, they are utilized as oxygen concentrators.

The air/oxygen blenders contain two separate gas lines. Each mixture is set at the same pressure of 50 psig. Whenever compressed air is delivered through a ventilator or other high pressure device, it's important to maintain the pressure above 30 psig. When the pressure decreases, an alarm sounds. Check for excessive condensation. Take the necessary steps to restore the pressure to make sure the proper oxygen blend is being delivered. If mechanical ventilation fails, be prepared to manually deliver oxygen to the patient until the system is restored.

Venturi mask

Venturi masks are used for patients with irregular breathing patterns. Variable breathing patterns cause uncertain changes in the I: E ratio, and minute volume. Control of the oxygen percentage with the Venturi mask allows the patient's needs to be more adequately met than with other oxygen delivery devices. The Venturi mask entrains (catches) room air. It is necessary to deliver oxygen flow rates that are four to six times the measured minute volume for this type of patient. To adjust the flow, look at the following: 5L of O2 is delivered through the Venturi mask and the minute volume changes from 10 to 18L/min. A 30% Venturi mask is being used. This Venturi mask provides a ratio of 8:1, making the total ratio 9. The liter flow is 5. The minute volume is 18. Multiply 9 (ratio) x 5(liter flow) =45L/min. To provide four times the minute volume the liter flow must be adjusted. Adjusting the flow to 8L/min. will provide four times the measured minute volume, or 72L/min. (9x8=72). The oxygen percentage should be re- measured following adjustments.

Oxygen tent therapy

Oxygen tents are used for children who don't fit under a hood or who are active and won't stay under the oxygen hood. Croupy children are placed in an oxygen tent because the tent is cooled providing the needed treatment for croup. Cooling allows climate control by preventing heat from accumulating in the tent. Obtain a tent and an oxygen analyzer with probe. Place the probe level with the patient's nose. Set up the nebulizer to keep the humidity greater than or at 60%. Set up the oxygen flow meter and set it at 8-10 or 12-15L/min. You will need to keep 35-50% oxygen in the tent, so the flow depends on whether the tent is small or large. Keep the tent sealed and tucked under the mattress to prevent oxygen escape. Toys that could induce spark (electric, battery) should not enter the tent due to fire hazard. Check oxygen delivery with an analyzer. Set the nebulizer accordingly and use the entrainment ports on the nebulizer to adjust to the desire oxygen level.

Oxygen concentrators

Oxygen concentrators are designed for home use because they provide low flow, continuous oxygen. Many people prefer to use small, portable devices that combine the oxygen tank and the compressor. Molecular-sieve concentrators deliver higher oxygen percentages. The flow rate must be adjusted when using a molecular sieve concentrator, to provide the correct oxygen percentage. The following provides flow/oxygen percentages delivered with the molecular sieve concentrator:

- 1-2L/min=> 90%
- 3-5L/min= 80-90%
- 6L/min= approx. 75%
- 8L/min= approx. 60%
- 10L/min= 50%

Higher flow rates deliver less oxygen percentage because more room air is "sifted" through the oxygen canisters removing more oxygen, nitrogen and water vapor. Permeable plastic membrane units pull air and water through the membrane, come with a condenser system and provide humidity. When using a permeable plastic membrane unit the flow can be set a 1-10L/min. but the oxygen percentage is fixed at 40%.

Oxygen hoods

Oxygen tents and oxygen hoods are similar because they provide a controlled environment for humidified, controlled oxygenation. An oxygen hood is used for infants who weigh no more than eighteen pounds. It is more desirable than a tent because it allows better access to patient care. Oxygen hoods provide a warm environment as opposed to the cooling mist provided to an oxygen tent. The humidifier must be warmed to the body temperature of the infant and monitored at all times by placing a thermometer inside the hood. The infant's temperature must be monitored regularly. The hood should remain sealed to prevent oxygen escape. Obtain the humidifier and warm it to the proper temperature. Use an air/oxygen proportioner and a flow meter and set it to at least 7L/min. Higher flow may be needed to stabilize the oxygen percentage. Have an oxygen analyzer available for continuous use and place the probe level with the infant's nose. It is possible to damage the infant's hearing, so care is taken to avoid noise above 65 decibels when working within the hood.

Oxygen conserving nasal cannula

Oxygen conserving cannulas are used with patients who require long term oxygen therapy. They are cost effective because they can be combined with an oxygen delivery device that delivers oxygen in timed doses. Oxygen conserving cannulas work by way of a reservoir. When the patient exhales, the reservoir is filled. With inhalation, a dose of oxygen is delivered. Teaching involves that care be taken if the reservoir refuses to fill. Replacement is necessary if this happens because it means the diaphragm has failed. When it is functioning correctly the diaphragm moves in and out. Two types of reservoirs are used with oxygen conserving cannulas. One type incorporates the reservoir into the cannula. The other type of conserving reservoir is incorporated into the oxygen tubing so that it hangs at chest level.

Ultrasonic nebulizer

When the unit is set up properly, installed and connected to the electrical outlet you should see ultrasonic activity in the chamber and aerosol is visible. Fill the fluid to the proper levels. No aerosol will be dispensed if the level is low. Read the directions from the manufacturer to ensure that set up is done properly. Problems can occur if the nebulizer chamber is not clean, if the water is too cold, if the power source is missing or if air leaks are present. Make sure to flush the system, make sure the unit is clean and that your power source is working. Ultrasonic units produce higher output of aerosol so they provide nebulization to the small airways. The unit delivers the aerosol by way of a built in fan.

Pneumatic nebulizer

Use a pneumatic nebulizer when it is necessary to change the patient's inspired oxygen percentage. The jet is powered by oxygen so the ports can be open if the oxygen percentage needs to be reduced. Close the ports to increase the oxygen percentage. You can provide 35-100% inspired oxygen with a pneumatic nebulizer. The oxygen is provided through a flow meter. The flow meter is adjusted to control the amount of aerosol. The particle size is more uniform because the liquid is dispensed against a baffle. The liquid flows up to the jet to provide nebulization and oxygen as opposed to bubble humidifiers where the oxygen flows downward into the capillary tube. Check the equipment to make sure the water level is correct. Capillary and large tubing must be kept clear of condensation. Water in the aerosol tube increases the percent of inspired oxygen by increasing pressure on the jet. Check that all parts are included and that assembly is correct before treatment is started.

Mainstream and sidestream nebulizers

Mainstream and sidestream nebulizers are examples of small volume nebulizers. As with other nebulizers, they are aerosolized with either air or oxygen. Mainstream nebulizers provide medication and gas directly to the patient. A separate gas powered jet is used to supply the aerosol. The sidestream nebulizer delivers the aerosol from the main gas flow. Most of the units are hand held, disposable and can be used with IPPB circuits. Particle filters are available for use to minimize any ill effects of aerosol as it escapes into the air. It is possible to inadvertently deliver medication to the therapist or caregivers. A one way valve can also be attached. To generate aerosol flow, delivery must be adequate and at least 3ml of solution should be contained in the reservoir.

Laryngoscope

Laryngoscopes and the accompanying blades are found on the hospital crash cart. There are several types of laryngoscope blades. The plastic or stainless steel handle is separate. Choose the type of blade then snap it to the laryngoscope handle to check the light source. If the light doesn't come on, check the handle for tight connection and check the bulb. Laryngoscopes on hospital crash carts are subject to routine inspection for proper operation. When the light source is dim, replace the batteries. Bulbs should be readily available for replacement. Either a curved or straight and curved blade can be used to intubate. The type of blade used is usually just a matter of preference. Pediatric and adult blades can be curved or straight. The straight blade is called a Miller, curved is a MacIntosh blade. Proper operation and use of the laryngoscope is vital during endotracheal intubation.

Pneumotachometer

The pneumotachometer is used to perform bedside spirometry. It converts lung measurements into an electrical signal for analysis. It is used to measure airflow during pulmonary function studies. Testing is done before and after a bronchodilator is given. The Fleisch pneumotachometer makes use of a pressure transducer to calculate the results. Heated pneumotachometers contain a heated wire. When gas is passes through, the heat is diminished. The amount of electrical energy used to keep the heat constant is used to measure the amount of gas flow. The devices must be properly calibrated to deliver accurate results. Several efforts from the patient are obtained and the highest result is used.

Coude catheter

The Coude catheter has a curved tip to allow suctioning of either the right or left bronchus. The anatomy of the adult tends to frequently lead a straight catheter into the right main stem bronchus. The Coude catheter lets you target the patient's needs more easily. The patient with right sided pneumonia will have increased secretions on the right, making this type of catheter a better choice. Pick a catheter that is less than ½ the diameter of the inside of the endotracheal tube. Suction the patient only when clinically indicated or as specifically directed by the physician. Recommend changes based on the physical assessment of the patient. Use the lowest level of vacuum necessary during suctioning.

Bird for IPPB

After you check the gas source and regulator, attach the hose and the IPPB unit to the source. Use your judgment regarding the delivery of humidity during the treatment. Look at the equipment carefully to make sure all the connections are tight. Depending on the patient's diagnosis, you may want to use the bacterial filter. The filter is placed between the gas outlets and the nebulizer hoses. Turn the unit on and let it cycle after you've set the pressure, flow and sensitivity. You can watch the machine cycle by placing your hand over the mouthpiece. Make sure there is a mist, and then add medication to the nebulizer. The large hose connects to the right side of the Bird unit and the other to the nebulizer. The small hose connects to a small opening on the right side of the unit and the other to a T piece at the nebulizer. A portion of the small tube is then used to connect one end of the T-piece with the exhalation valve.

Backpressure compensated flowmeters

Backpressure compensated flow meters have the flow control valve below the meter. As gas is delivered upward these types of flowmeters, provide very accurate readings. They are the most desirable devices to indicate proper oxygen flow, but only in the upright position. Turn on the meter and look for the liter flow indicator (ball) to bounce. These types of meters cannot be laid flat because the back pressure will provide an incorrect reading. The respiratory therapist is responsible for quality controls on respiratory equipment. In order to check for correct oxygen delivery you should provide a known oxygen flow through the meter, performed with the meter upright. If there is a question about proper function, the equipment should be replaced and removed from the patient care area for repair. Follow the protocol at your institution to report inoperable equipment.

Infection control

Wash your hands before and after patient contact, when you start your shift, and when you are leaving the workplace. Wear a gown, gloves and protective eyewear when indicated. It's important to assess the patient to determine the equipment required to prevent contamination from airborne bacteria, sputum, blood and other body fluid contamination. Dispose of all biohazardous materials properly. For known or suspected tuberculosis, a special, properly fitted mask must be worn. This is mandated by the National Institute of Occupational Safety and Health. If you are ill, have an infection, open cuts, rashes or skin irritations you should not provide direct patient care. Follow all guidelines that are hospital specific. Never try to recap a needle. Sputum, blood cultures and other specimens must be contained securely and placed in a bag marked for the laboratory. If blood or body fluids are spilled, follow hospital procedure and immediately have the area cleaned Try to avoid mouth to mouth resuscitation; use a mouth to valve mask. Report any incidence of self contamination and follow institutional guidelines for decontamination.

Retard exhalation

Retard exhalation capabilities exist when providing IPPB. Depending which machine you are using, either a valve or cap can be used. Retard exhalation is used to prevent over inflation of the lungs. It provides the pressure needed to keep the small airways open longer so that more air can be released during exhalation. The amount necessary is based on the measurement of the exhaled volumes during the treatment. Decide how much retard to apply by asking the patient how he feels. Note if he is able to completely release the delivered tidal volume. Too much resistance increases intrathoracic pressure. The patient may feel uncomfortable by the increased amount of time it takes to breathe out. Remember that with IPPB, tidal volume delivery is controlled by adjusting the peak pressure.

Heat moisture exchanger

Heat moisture exchangers (HMEs) allow the patient to breathe warm moist air. They are assembled and ready for use. Each exhaled breath is warmed and moistened by the unit. The units are disposable and can be replaced if they become inoperable from damage or from obstruction by patient secretions. Heat moisture exchangers can be applied to a tracheostomy tube during mechanical ventilation and when patients are breathing independently. During mechanical ventilation, the HME is attached to the patient and to the ventilator circuit. Patients who are not mechanically ventilated have the HME attached to the airway. The other end is open to room air. Patients with a permanent tracheostomy can carry a heat moisture exchanger with them if needed.

High frequency airway oscillation

A device with a vibrating flutter valve can be used to provide high frequency oscillation. It is usually used following medication administration and is especially useful for patients with cystic fibrosis. The device resembles a pipe with a steel ball in it that flutters, providing oscillation and movement of secretions. Flutter valve devices are preassembled and ready for use. Some have adjustable settings to adjust the pressures and frequency of oscillation. Demonstrate deep comfortable breathing. Show the patient how to exhale through the mouthpiece. Treatment should be performed for about twenty minutes using intervals of 10 – 20 breaths followed by coughing after each series of inhalation and exhalations. Each time the breathing exercises are repeated more pressure is exerted on the airway. Stop the treatment if it becomes uncomfortable for the patient and recommend an alternative treatment.

Bag valve mask device

The ambu bag or bag valve mask device is used to provide ventilatory support during CPR, periods of extended apnea and whenever a patient who is not breathing requires oxygenation or resuscitation. The bag valve mask contains a self inflating bag, or reservoir that is connected to a high flow oxygen source. A one way valve is present to prevent rebreathing and provide positive pressure to the airways. Various sizes are available for neonates, children and adults to deliver the proper amount of volume from the reservoir. Pediatric ambu bags have a pop off valve to adjust the pressure and prevent lung injury. The various reservoirs contain 250-500ml for infants and children and 1500-2000ml for adults. The bag is easily fitted to an artificial airway for use. During manual resuscitation it is important to make sure the patient's oxygen mask is tightly fitted and that chest movement is seen when the reservoir is activated.

Minute ventilation

When using minute ventilation to adjust blood gases, increase the minute ventilation to improve oxygenation. Once the patient's tidal volume and respiratory rates are maximized, look at the minute ventilation to make sure it is also adequate to meet the patient's oxygen demands. Adjustment of PCO2 is accomplished by adjusting tidal volume, then respiratory rate. To further modify ventilation to the alveoli, adjust the minute ventilation. Use of the following formula should be helpful:

PaCO2 (*current) x VE

PaCO2 (*desired CO2 level)

Once the minute volume change is determined it can be applied by reducing tidal volume. The respiratory rate can also be reduced to decrease the minute volume. It should be kept in mind that minute volumes are more stable than the tidal volume and are considered important for this reason when making adjustments during mechanical ventilation.

Quality-Control

Liquid oxygen safety

Liquid oxygen units allow patient mobility, are cost effective and don't require cylinder changes. A reservoir is kept in the home for oxygen refill. Safety regulations are in place for home use of liquid oxygen and the respiratory therapist should know how to properly set up a liquid oxygen system and properly instruct the patient and family. It is mandatory to avoid contact with liquid oxygen. If this occurs, medical treatment is necessary. If a spill occurs, wait 15 minutes before cleaning the area and wear insulated gloves to avoid skin contact. No smoking signs must be displayed in the home and heating sources near the unit must be avoided. Frostbite occurs when liquid oxygen contacts the skin. Goggles, high top boots, and insulated gloves must be worn when filling from the oxygen reservoir. Nothing that could cause ignition should be within five feet of the oxygen unit. Proper placement and stabilization of the unit at all times will prevent tipping and fire hazard. It is the respiratory therapist's responsibility to maintain and troubleshoot home oxygen equipment.

Quality control for blood gas analyzers

Quality control measures are performed on the electrodes for PO_2, PCO_2 and PH. Quality control measure must be accurate and documented. The system must be properly calibrated. Several different materials are used depending on the equipment at your facility. Any time quality control measures deviate from the standard it means the equipment is out of control and the situation much be investigated. When an error is found, the control measure should be repeated. Become familiar with the specification on the blood gas analyzer. Learn to troubleshoot problems by reading the manufacturer's recommendations. To predict PCO_2 at a given CO_2 or O_2 percentage you will need the following equation:

$$PCO_2 \text{ or } O_2 = (Pb - PH_2O \text{ x } \%CO_2 \text{ or } O_2.$$

Therapeutic procedure initiation and modification

Therapies

Respiratory care

Assess your patient before, during and after respiratory therapy interventions. Recommend changes in the treatment plan based on your assessment. If your patient is not meeting measurable goals according to the plan you have established you should work with other team member to develop a new plan. Set a time for your patient to meet goals and document your conversations and assessment after each interaction with your patient. Take part in discharge planning. Make certain the patient will be able to financially and physically comply with his medical regimen. Educate your patient to facilitate a complete understanding of his respiratory ailment. This is especially important for patients with asthma and COPD. Use community and written resources to find ways to help your patient comprehend the disease process. Include family members in the teaching. Identify all sources of patient support and discuss areas of concern with the physician.

Chest percussion

Chest percussion is used to provide pulmonary hygiene to mobilize secretions and clear the airways. Focus is on the area with secretions. Use one or both hands to cup the chest while the patient is placed with his head down or sitting in a chair. The position of the patient will depend on the area being targeted. The chair position is used to target the lower portion of the upper lobes of the lungs, while the patient's back is toward the therapist. Cupping of the hands is done to entrap air and as the hands are removed a startling sound is produced; a "pop". Devices to percuss the chest are available for infants and adults. When percussing the chest of an infant manually, use the first three fingers in a curved fashion to cover the smaller amount of surface area. Provide percussion therapy for 1 to 5 minutes, according to the tolerance of the patient. Discontinue the treatment if the patient develops discomfort or respiratory distress. Percussion as a part pulmonary hygiene is combined with postural drainage and vibration.

PEEP

PEEP is Positive End Expiratory Pressure and is used to prevent alveolar collapse. It is a pressure set above that of normal atmosphere and it provides maintenance of FRC (functional residual capacity). PEEP is used in conjunction with oxygen administration to facilitate the lowest use of oxygen delivery. The goal is to maintain PaO2 greater than 60 and O2 sat >90%. CPAP has a similar effect. A general rule is that if your patient is receiving too much PEEP and develops hypotension or decreased cardiac output you should decrease PEEP. Conversely, PEEP may need to be increased in hypoxic states and when oxygen requirements are 50% or higher. PEEP is commonly used in any condition where FRC is diminished.

PEEP should be applied carefully. Start with low levels, evaluate the patient and increase PEEP levels 2-5cm. at a time until the patient's respiratory status is optimized. Too much PEEP reduces cardiac output and the symptoms include tachycardia, hypotension and low in Pvo2. Subcutaneous emphysema, pneumothorax and pulmonary interstitial emphysema are complications. Though PEEP increases FRC and is valuable in treating ARDS, atelectasis as well as pulmonary edema the respiratory therapist must be aware of the possibility of untoward effects. When patient goals are met, it is important to begin the process of decreasing the amount of PEEP. This is especially true when higher levels (10-15cm.H20) are necessary to reduce pulmonary shunting. Since oxygen toxicity can occur, PEEP is used to reduce the need for high oxygen flows. Monitor the patient closely and withdraw PEEP according to your patient's measured response; when oxygenation is at or >60torr, oxygen delivery is in the mid range, if instability occurs indicative of decreased cardiac output, or if barotrauma becomes evident.

CPAP

CPAP is similar to PEEP. The main differences between the two are that the patient must be adequately breathing and CPAP is less likely to affect cardiac output, allowing for higher levels of pressure. Otherwise, the uses and benefits are the same. CPAP can be adjusted according to the carbon dioxide measurement to treat hypoxemia. If there is any indication that mechanical ventilation might be required CPAP should not be initiated. Monitor for signs of fatigue and adjust CPAP when CO2 levels are low or hypoxemia is present. If maximum levels of CPAP are being used and hypoxemia is persistent, the patient must be mechanically ventilated. Note the workload of breathing by assessing for complaints of dyspnea and use of accessory muscles of respiration. If vital signs are not stable, or become unstable CPAP should not be used.

IPPB

IPPB is useful in a variety of settings. It is used to facilitate the expectoration of sputum, treat respiratory failure during hypoventilation, decrease venous return to the heart in the treatment of CHF, and is used to deliver medications. AARC guidelines state that IPPB is never to be used in the presence of pneumothorax. IPPB can lead to a tension pneumothorax. After a tension pneumothorax has been treated with chest tube insertion, IPPB can be considered. Caution should be exercised for patients with head injury or increased intracranial pressure, tuberculosis, esophageal surgery, face, head neck or throat surgery, fistulas of the trachea/esophagus, hemoptysis or who are hemodynamically unstable. Any patient with increased airway resistance can experience over inflation of the alveoli resulting in air trapping. Extra care is taken in the presence of barotrauma, very thick secretions, and infection that is hospital acquired. Hyperventilation, hypocarbia, and gastric distention are possible adverse outcomes. Check to make sure the nebulizer is secure. A bacterial filter should always be present when the patient is being treated for infection.

Before administering IPPB, review the orders. Gather and assemble the IPPB equipment and medication before you enter the patient's room. Explain the procedure and identify that you are the respiratory therapist. Check the ID bracelet. Interview the patient and do a physical assessment. IPPB units either require electricity or compressed air to operate. Set the parameters, set the prescribed oxygen flow, and adjust the peak pressure to 10-15cm.H20 and -1 cm. H2O pressure. The nebulizer should be set to run on inspiration. Turn on the machine to make sure it is operating properly. Instruct the patient to relax and let the machine fill the lungs. When the lungs are full, have the patient hold his breath for 2-3 seconds then exhale slowly. When giving an active treatment, instruct the patient to inhale deeply and use peak pressures according to the patient's tolerance. There are several types of IPPB machines available.   Become familiar with the equipment at your institution. Check for air leaks around the patient's mouth, in the circuitry or in the tracheal or endotracheal cuff if the IPPB machine fails to cycle.

Oxygen therapy risks

Oxygen is a medication. Complaints of dyspnea don't always require oxygen administration, such as dyspnea that is the result of hyperventilation during an anxiety attack. Blood gas analysis provides definitive information to guide treatment. You must have a doctor's order to administer oxygen, except during CPR, a heart attack, or when a patient is bleeding or severely hypotensive. PO2 levels should be kept at 50 to 60% (torr). CO2 retention from hyperoxygenation will lead to hypoventilation. Atelectasis can result from increased oxygen uptake by hemoglobin. Providing more than 80% oxygen leads to alveolar collapse. Oxygen toxicity is believed to occur at levels greater than 50%. If more oxygen is required, it must be limited to less than 72 hours. Infants born prematurely will develop retinopathy and blindness if high levels of oxygen are administered.

Heliox and nitric oxide therapy

Administering Heliox, (oxygen and helium), is an effective treatment for obstructive airway disease. It is used to reduce airway resistance, decreasing the work of breathing. Helium is less dense than air. The mixture is given with a non-rebreathing mask. Helium concentrated with 20, 30 or 40% oxygen can be used, depending on the written order. You must adjust the oxygen flow meter when using Heliox. Adjustment is made by dividing the observed flow by the Heliox factor. Example: 60%Helium/40%oxygen = 1:4 Heliox factor - Using 6L/min. x 1.4 = 8.4L/min. actual flow.

Nitric oxide is primarily administered to treat persistent pulmonary hypertension and RDS in newborns. It has also been used to treat adults with pulmonary hypertension and ARDS. Nitric oxide dilates the pulmonary blood vessels and is delivered through a ventilator. The INOVvent system is used to set the desired concentration of oxygen and nitric oxide. It can also be delivered manually, or with a resuscitator when necessary.

Tracheostomy

Tracheostomy tubes can be temporary or permanent. Tracheostomy is usually performed in the operating room. Provision of an artificial airway through the trachea allows for long term airway and short term management following surgery or head, neck and facial trauma. Tracheostomy tubes are used to prevent aspiration when a patient cannot swallow. Patients who are unable to wean from the ventilator will likely receive a tracheostomy to prevent complications from prolonged intubation. A tracheostomy allows the patient to eat and drink and is more comfortable than an endotracheal tube. Other indications include coma, tumors, and congenital defects of the trachea or larynx.

Proper tracheostomy care is aimed toward the prevention of mucous plugs by providing humidity of 100%. The tracheostomy tube is changed routinely after the initial healing. Infection control includes keeping the site of the tracheostomy clean and dry. Ongoing attention is given to proper cuff pressure to prevent arterial or tracheal fistula. Emergency tracheostomy change may be required if respiratory distress if present. Suction first and if resistance is encountered during suctioning the tube must be replaced.

When changing a tracheostomy tube, wear goggles, gloves and a gown. Change the tracheostomy tube using sterile technique. Check the tube size and have one size smaller available. Obtain the inner cannula, tracheostomy tubes, normal saline to clean, ties to secure the outer cannula, a precut gauze pad, sterile utensils, sterile gloves, an obturator and water soluble lubricant, such as KY jelly. Use a 10cc. syringe for the cuff. Prelubricate the tracheostomy tube and have your equipment open and ready to use, maintaining sterile technique. Explain the procedure. Make sure the obturator fits easily into the tracheostomy tube. Deflate the cuff. Cut the ties and remove the tracheostomy tube carefully. Have the fresh tube ready to insert. Pre oxygenate the patient, and then suction the trachea. Clean the area around the stoma with sterile saline and dry it well. Put in the new tube using the obturator. It should glide easily. Do not force it. Remove the guide, place the inner cannula and lock it into place. Inflate the cuff, place the clean gauze and secure with the ties. Assess breath sounds.

Fenestrated tracheostomy tube and tracheostomy button
A fenestrated tracheostomy allows the patient to breathe through the fenestrated opening when the tracheostomy tube is plugged. It is used in anticipation of removing the standard tracheostomy tube in a patient who is breathing spontaneously. The outer cannula blocks the patient's airflow when it is plugged, and allows breathing through the hole, or fenestration.

The tracheostomy button covers the patient's tracheotomy stoma to keep it open following tracheostomy tube removal. It is a safety measure to provide airway access during recovery. The device consists of an inner and outer cannula. The inner cannula is held in place by a flange that keeps it from being easily coughed out. Spacers keep the stoma open and are used to keep the button in the proper position. A special button is available for exhalation only that allows the patient to speak. Make sure the size of the button is the same as the tracheostomy tube.

Tracheal cuff volume

Cuff pressure should be as low as possible to prevent erosion and vascular damage. Most patients will require no more than 15mm/Hg cuff pressure, but the patient's blood pressure must be taken into consideration. If blood pressure is low, there is less capillary pressure to protect the trachea. When the patient is hypertensive, more resistance can be tolerated because the blood flow to the area is greater, lessening the chance of vascular compromise. Check the pressure every eight hours. Use the initial documentation for comparison. If cuff pressure exceeds the recommended maximum, discuss it with the physician. The tracheostomy tube may need to be replaced. Observe for signs of tracheal erosion by observing secretions. Report any signs of bleeding.

Endotracheal extubation

Measure the patient's pulmonary status and make certain the minimum requirements have been met. Inform the patient what you're going to do and explain how it will feel. Instruct the patient to cough following removal of the tube and place the patient in optimal position. Suction and then oxygenate the patient. Many therapists apply suction during removal of the tube. Endotracheal suctioning is a sterile procedure. The patient is always hyperoxygenated prior to suctioning with 100% 02. Provide a sigh breath then deflate the cuff, pulling the tube out when the patient has received a full inhalation. Assist with coughing. After extubation, oxygenate the patient at the previous settings using aerosol. Recheck ABG's in 20-30 minutes. SP02 should be continuously monitored and care is taken to have the patient take frequent deep breaths. Observe for laryngospasm and edema. Racemic epinephrine is may be necessary if airway edema becomes evident. Report bleeding and watch for vocal cord paralysis.

PEP

PEP is positive expiratory pressure therapy. PEP therapy is used to minimize air trapping and helps reduce carbon dioxide levels in patients with emphysema. Pressure is applied to the airways through a mask or mouthpiece to prevent atelectasis. PEP is also used to treat atelectasis and provides therapy to patients over age four with cystic fibrosis. Aerosolized medications can be delivered during PEP therapy to maximize the effect of bronchodilators. Various types of equipment are available for use. The respiratory therapy should learn to properly assemble the device and learn how to troubleshoot problems. PEP should not be used after trauma or surgery to the upper body. Patients with increased ICP are at risk for worsening when PEP is applied. Any active bleeding from the lungs or nose is a contraindication. If the patient is nauseated, PEP may induce vomiting. Discontinue the treatment if the patient develops respiratory distress, or complains of chest pain (PEP increases the work of the heart). Make certain that the device is well fitted to your patient and be aware that PEP can cause trauma.

Differential lung ventilation

Situations exist that require each lung to be separately ventilated. Examples include injury to one lung, pneumonia, ARDS and after thoracic surgery. Some esophageal surgeries, pulmonary embolism, fistula and lung transplant may also require separate lung ventilation. A double lumen endotracheal tube is used to manage separate ventilators. Synchronous breathing is possible by adjusting separate tidal volumes, FIO2 and PEEP. The tidal volume is set to ½ the normal patient standard for the functioning lung while the injured or healing lung receives little tidal volume. If an air leak is present from a fistula the injured lung would require lower settings while the fistula is allowed to heal and synchronized breathing is not possible. As the patient progresses, a change can be made to normal ventilation by using an adaptor. Close observation of blood gas analysis is required. When lung compliance is equal in both lungs, conventional ventilation is initiated. It is important to regulate peak pressure to allow healing of the lung. A single lumen endotracheal tube should be used once the patient improves.

Management of Hypoxia and hypercapnia

In order to manage hypoxia you must determine the cause and try different ventilator modes. Hypoxemia from ARDS and shunting may respond to increased FIO2 or CPAP. PEEP should also be considered. Measure the PaO2, lung compliance, vital signs, PVR, and cardiac output to identify therapy outcomes. If the PaO2 improves, but cardiac output falls a change of therapy is needed.

In the case of hypercapnia, the cause must be reviewed. If the patient has worsening COPD, consider using MMV ventilation. During the withdrawal of neuromuscular blocking agents or sedation, MMV mode may be beneficial. The minute volume is delivered according to the clinical condition. Other approaches include switching to AC ventilator mode or control. Once the patient is stable, it should be possible to switch to IMV or SIMV mode in preparation for weaning.

Pulmonary rehabilitation

Evaluate the patient's present level of activity. Assess lifestyle habits and set realistic goals. Observe the patient during activity. Document the patient's abilities by describing symptoms, how frequently the patient stops activity to rest, and the results of the pulse oximeter before and after walking. Involve the patient's physician and family in assisting with lifestyle changes, such as weight loss and smoking cessation and proper nutrition. Ongoing education is necessary. Encourage enrollment in a formal pulmonary rehabilitation program. Be familiar the patient's record for vital signs, pulmonary function tests, and blood test results. Suggest studies that may have not been performed. The respiratory therapist should be aware of the benefits of exercise and discuss these benefits thoroughly with the patient. Emphasize the fact that the patient is likely to be hospitalized less. An individualized exercise program will include strength and endurance training. Encourage patient feedback and perform ongoing assessment. Provide input for the patient regarding gains or needed areas of improvement. Listen to how the patient perceives rehabilitation efforts. Communicate with team members and recommend changes as needed.

Bronchoscopy

Bronchoscopy is performed to diagnosis lung disorders, remove bronchial secretions and to treat aspiration. Also, it is used to remove mucous plugs, perform biopsy, treat severe hemoptysis, remove foreign bodies, obtain sputum for pathology, and assess for injury. Two types of bronchoscopes can be employed, flexible or rigid. The flexible bronchoscope is referred to as a fiberoptic bronchoscope. Use of the rigid bronchoscope can induce or otherwise promote existing lung injury. Because the scope is not flexible, it cannot be placed beyond the right or left main stem bronchus. Close observation of the patient is necessary during the procedure. Adequate oxygenation must be maintained. Observe for cardiac arrhythmias. If tissue is sampled bleeding may occur. The patient should have a stable cardiac status to reduce the risk of M.I. Transbronchial bronchoscopy can result in damage to the trachea.

Chest tube insertion

The most emergent need for a chest tube is tension pneumothorax. Rapid lung expansion is performed by inserting a large bore needle into the chest to quickly remove air and decrease pressure on the heart and blood vessels. The needle is inserted emergently and temporarily, followed by a chest tube. Chest tubes are used to remove air and blood from the pleural space and to treat cardiac tamponade. Air and blood found in the mediastinal space is removed with chest tube drainage. Purulence from empyema may require drainage. Set up the chest tube drainage system on the right or left, depending on the need. Expose the affected lung by turning the patient. After the tube is inserted by the physician using sterile technique, it is secured with sutures and sterile dressing is applied. Maintain wall suction to the drainage system. Observe for bubbling in the drainage system. Measure liquid drainage and record it. Keep all the connections secure. If changes occur suddenly, notify the physician. Obtain a Chest X-Ray. Monitor the patient closely.

Aerosol tent

The aerosol tent is set up just as an oxygen tent. Instead of oxygen, compressed air is piped into the tent through a nebulizer. The aerosol tent is used for children with croup or laryngotracheobronchitis. Most children are too active to wear an aerosol mask. The tent should be filled with at least 10L/min of air. Cooling mist is required to help reduce airway edema. The top of the tent should be opened to avoid carbon dioxide buildup and fogginess while still providing aerosol. Use a mask when possible to deliver aerosol. Remember that aerosol can cause bronchospasm. Listen for new development of wheezing whenever aerosol is being delivered. Aerosol should not be used long term in the newborn due avoid fluid overload.

Aerosol considerations

Particle size should be considered when providing aerosol treatments. Larger particles treat the upper airways. The alveoli are treated with smaller particles. Lower flow rates deliver smaller particles. Slower inhalation ensures better delivery of medication to lower airways. If possible, the patient should wait ten seconds before exhaling. To deliver aerosol to the upper airways the patient should be instructed to breathe at a normal rate and pattern. The flow should be high. Various nebulizers deliver different sized aerosol particles. High frequency ultrasonic nebulizers can deliver smaller particle size and high flow to the lower airways but carry the risk of bronchospasm, medication breakdown, and overhydration. The smaller particles are due to the high frequency. Ultrasonic nebulizers use sterile water which is more irritating than normal saline. Small volume ultrasonic nebulizers can be used for mechanically ventilated patients but they are large and cumbersome.

TTO

Transtracheal oxygen (TTO) can be delivered directly to the trachea with a flexible hollow catheter. Patients with COPD and long term oxygen use benefit from this type of oxygen delivery. A puncture is made into the trachea, just large enough to accommodate the catheter. It is performed as an outpatient and is a short procedure. The patient benefits by using less oxygen. The delivery of oxygen through the catheter is less conspicuous as wearing a nasal cannula. Nasal irritation is avoided. The puncture site heals readily if the patient no longer desires to use it. The patient is instructed how to change the catheter tubing and how to flush it with saline to keep it patent. Many patients experience increased exercise capacity with TTO delivery. Oxygen costs are lower due to the lower settings. If the catheter becomes plugged, nasal oxygen can be used by the patient.

MDI

MDI is the abbreviation for metered dose inhaler. Metered dose inhalers propel a measured amount of medication to the lungs from a pressurized chamber. The inhaler is primed according to the amount of medication prescribed. Each time the inhaler is activated the amount of medication is increased, or the dose can be delivered in serial inhalations. Bronchodilators, steroids and antibiotics are commonly dispensed with MDI's. The patient turns the inhaler over to fill the chamber with medication then places it to the mouth in the upright position to activate it while inhaling through the mouthpiece. MDI's can be used with an adaptor for patients who are intubated or during special procedures. Spacers are often used to deliver the medication more slowly and comfortably. The spacer must be cleaned after each use with a disinfectant or white vinegar.

Sigh volume

The upper level of VT in the adult patient who is mechanically ventilated is 15ml/kg of body weight. When CO2 levels become decreased it is necessary to decrease tidal volume.

The lower level is 10ml/kg body weight. Sigh volumes can be administered to provide the patient with extra tidal volume. Sighing is considered a physiologically normal occurrence; we sigh every few minutes. Sigh volumes are delivered in the A/C mode during mechanical ventilation. The respiratory therapist must determine what, if any benefits will be derived by the patient by increasing the rate and/or volume of sighs. Larger sigh volumes are indicated when the patient has atelectasis or segmental consolidation. However, if the tidal volume is at the upper limits, this may not be at all necessary. Consideration must be given to the use of sigh volume during mechanical ventilation. Weigh the benefits and look at the indications and contraindications. Patients who are sensitive to increased airway pressure or have air trapping should not receive sighs.

Inspiratory hold

Inspiratory hold is used to improve oxygenation in patients with decreased lung compliance (ARDS, pulmonary edema). It allows for more even distribution of tidal volume. When the patient is temporarily prevented from exhaling tidal volume, the lungs reach the inspiratory plateau. The longer the hold, the more oxygen is delivered throughout the lungs. Inspiratory plateau should not be added if the patient has normal lung compliance and adequate ventilation. Since the addition of inspiratory hold shortens the expiratory time, consideration is given to adjusting the I:E ratio. Close monitoring is needed to evaluate when the inspiratory hold can be decreased. Different ventilators measure inspiratory hold times depending on the manufacturer.

Expiratory retard

Expiratory retard is used to open the alveoli. This has been discussed relative to IPPB treatment. Some ventilators allow adjustments for inspiratory and expiratory retard. Expiratory retard is used during mechanical ventilation when the patient is unable to completely exhale due to air trapping, such as with COPD and asthma. Remember that the inspiratory and expiratory volumes should be the same when performing these measurements. When airway resistance is normal, expiratory retard should no longer be needed. When assessing breath sounds, listen as wheezing is diminished at the end of exhalation. There should be no pauses between exhalation and the beginning of the next inhalation. Further adjustments may be necessary if auto PEEP is detected. Close patient monitoring and adjustments followed by reassessment will help you determine the correct application of expiratory retard.

Emergency therapies

Mouth to mouth resuscitation

The first person who discovers a non breathing patient should perform mouth to mouth resuscitation. Review the techniques to open the airway. Make a good seal with your mouth. Pinch the adult's nose and block the nose of the infant with your mouth. Deliver two breaths, large enough to see the chest rise. Allow the person to exhale before giving the next breath. Use as little "force" as necessary as you observe the rise and fall of the chest, being especially cautious with infants and children. Adults should receive rescue breathing at 10-12 breaths per minute. Neonate rescue breathing is performed at a rate of 40-60 breaths per minute, and children 20 per minute. Allow six seconds between rescue breaths for adults, three seconds for children and about 1-1/2 seconds for the neonate will help you time the delivery. Remember that air can enter the stomach if too large a tidal volume is given.

Mouth to valve mask resuscitator

The mouth to valve resuscitator provides the rescuer with a barrier to the patient. Available sizes include infant, child and adult. There is a one way valve present to let the rescuer breathe into the patient's mouth effectively and provide life support. The mask and barrier must fit properly to prevent the escape of air during CPR or rescue breathing. A device that allows air to escape back into the rescuers mouth is not properly designed or is damaged. Double shield barriers are available that fit the patient's face, followed by a spacer and a second barrier. This type of device allows the rescuer to use the hand to keep the first shield sealed and the mask well anchored. The first barrier is flexible to allow escape of patient air each time the rescuers hands are released.

Home discharge

The respiratory therapist should be part of the discharge planning team. The family must be involved in teaching and support, especially if the patient is unable to perform activities of daily living. Use all of the most recent test results to assess the patient's capabilities. Be completely familiar with the disease process as you teach it to the patient and family. Become familiar with the layout of the home, presence of others who smoke whether the patient needs assistance with smoking cessation and what family support is readily available. Determine if the patient lives alone. Are family members close to the patient's home? Is there a spouse who can provide care? Are there modifications needed to the home such as ramps, or assistive devices? Determine the level of comprehension of the patient and family during teaching. Help your patient stop smoking. Nicotine replacement, such as Nicorette gum and nicotine patches can be purchased over the counter. Prescription medications are available and should be discussed with the physician. Support groups may be available to help.

Strength training exercises

The patient should have a targeted exercise routine aimed at strengthening large muscle groups. Debilitation lessens endurance, so strengthening is needed before other physical progress can be made. Focus on the arms, legs, abdomen and respiratory muscles. Provide instructions regarding warm up and cool down activities. Review basic stretching techniques and have the patient perform according to his or her individual capability. Have the patient use 1-2 pound weights for arm strengthening. This can even be done by using canned goods or barbell weights if available. Have the patient move the arms up, down, front and back while holding onto weights. Legs are exercised with weights placed on the ankles. Abdominal exercises are performed by placing the weight on the abdomen as the patient breathes against resistance. After strengthening exercises, walking or stretching should be performed again as a "cool down". Once the large muscles groups are strengthened, the patient can begin a more aerobic exercise program designed to increase metabolism.

Frequent patient turning and positioning

The patient who has a disease or has had surgery in one lung should be positioned so that the affected lung is in the upward position. This simple measure allows improved oxygenation and lung expansion. The patient with an artificial airway should be turned to keep secretions moving and to facilitate airway patency through proper alignment of the head and neck. Turning patients who are in a weakened state or who have pain helps in the prevention of atelectasis. Frequent turning facilitates circulation and patient comfort. It is also necessary to prevent skin breakdown and is mandatory to facilitate examination of your patient. Turn and position the patient for overall pulmonary hygiene. You will often find that after your patient is repositioned they will need suctioning. Don't forget to hyperoxygenate prior to suctioning. Remember to be cautious with patients who have active bleeding, neck injuries, head injuries, pleural effusions and anxiety with position changes. Be cautious with surgical incisions and pain control.

Patient concerns and therapist roles

Advanced directives, DNR and living will

Advanced directives, or a living will must be clearly stated and signed by the patient. Written directives must be clearly displayed on the patient's medical record. It is the responsibility of the healthcare team to uphold the patient's wishes regarding resuscitation and invasive medical therapies. The patient determines whether or not they wish to be supported on a ventilator, or receive CPR in the presence of terminal illness. The advanced directive from the patient that requests "No CPR" is commonly referred to as DNR, abbreviated from "do not resuscitate". Sometimes the decision to execute advanced

- 92 -

directives must be discussed with the patient by the healthcare team. When you are caring for a critically ill patient, in the hospital or in the home, become familiar with advanced directives that are already in place. Prepare to help the patient make decisions about a Living Will. The patient who expresses that their quality of life has become such that they no longer wish to receive medical treatment will need guidance and emotional support.

Respiratory therapist roles

If the physician has ordered postural drainage for your patient, you have reviewed the chart, and the nurse has documented that the patient's abdomen is distended and has turned off the patient's tube feedings, you should not perform postural drainage to a patient who has a distended abdomen. Until a diagnosis is made, there is a very real risk of aspiration. The patient who has abdominal distention will not tolerate being placed in Trendelenburg or reverse Trendelenburg position for pulmonary hygiene because of diaphragmatic interference with the lower lung segments. Document your findings on the chart and ask the physician to place the procedure on "hold" until further evaluation.

If you go to the patient's room to provide percussion and vibration and the patient complains of tenderness in the rib area. Discuss the patient's complaint with the physician and re-evaluate the appropriateness of the therapy when the patient's symptoms are resolved. Chest wall pain is a contraindication to performing percussion or vibration. If your patient is scheduled to receive postural drainage at 3pm and you find out that she has had a meal at 2:30 because she had been away from the room for special testing, postural drainage should not be provided within one hour of eating. Reschedule the therapy.

Neonatal and Infant Considerations

HFV in the neonate

HFV is used to treat the neonate who is not responding to conventional respiratory support. Respiratory rates up to 150/min. with a conventional ventilator can be used to deliver HFV. High respiratory rate settings are termed high frequency positive pressure ventilation (HFPV). True HFV is administered during high frequency oscillation (HFO) or by way of high frequency jet ventilation (HFJV) with a HFV ventilator. Jet ventilation directs small amounts of gas down the ET tube, traps additional gas and provides greater tidal volumes. Exhalation is passive during jet ventilation. An oscillator can be used to deliver small tidal volumes. Exhalation is active. The tidal volume is pulled from the lungs by backstroke of the piston in the oscillator. High frequency settings are 10-15 Hertz (one respiratory cycle per second). Increase or decrease the tidal volume by adjusting the jet pressure (drive pressure), or oscillator amplitude once the proper HFV is determined. Recommended uses for HFV include pneumomediastinum, pneumoperitoneum, pneumothorax, RDS, ARDS, bronchopleural fistula, air leak, PPHN, pulmonary hypoplasia and during tracheal, or bronchial surgery. HFV is used during bronchoscopy.

Infant apnea monitoring

Infants who experience periods of apnea may require home apnea monitoring. Explain the need to the parents. Premature infants have underdeveloped central nervous systems which affects breathing. Apnea monitoring is always recommended when there have been two or more incidences of SIDS death in the home or when the newborn has been in NICU. It's important for the family to understand the indications for apnea monitoring. How to set the alarms to alert the parents if the heart rate drops or if apnea occurs for >20 seconds. Two electrodes are placed somewhere on the infant's chest, abdomen, rib area or lower ribs. Proper electrode placement is performed to target the area where the greatest amount of respiratory movement is seen. Set the alarm to alert the parents to a decrease

<90% SpO2. Monitors that have a heart rate alarm should be set if the rate falls below 100. Have the family demonstrate use of the device and provide written instructions. The family should learn infant CPR.

CPAP delivery in newborns

CPAP is delivered nasally in newborns. CPAP is used to prevent endotracheal intubation with RDS or premature birth. CPAP forces air into the stomach. Make sure the nasogastric tube is working properly to avoid gastric reflux and aspiration. Become familiar with the CPAP unit. Increase flow if CPAP level decreases during inspiration by more than two centimeters. Observe the respiratory mechanics of the infant during CPAP. Observe breathing. If exhalation becomes an effort, the CPAP may be too high. If retractions are present, increase the flow. Check for mucous plugs and suction as needed. Check the respiratory rate, SPO2 and PaO2 levels. Check for proper assembly of the equipment, making sure that all tubes are patent. If CPAP falls to 0, the breathing circuit should be reassembled. Most likely, a break in the system has occurred. Provide manual ventilation while the system status is checked.

The use of CPAP and mechanical ventilation in infants requires close assessment. If CPAP has been discontinued due to low PaO2 or hypercarbia, mechanical ventilation may have been necessary. The goal is to wean the infant safely when PaO2 levels are improved on PEEP. Weaning from mechanical ventilation to CPAP is the normal procedure. In other words, ventilatory support includes CPAP or mechanical ventilation depending on the clinical situation and it may be necessary to switch from one to the other. During weaning, check the blood gas and vital signs. Keep the PaO2 50-70torr and add CPAP while you continue monitoring. If maximum CPAP is reached mechanical ventilation is again indicated. Decrease CPAP and oxygen delivery as the infant improves. CPAP may not be tolerated and should be initiated at 4-5cm.H20 pressure and increased by 2cm. Remember that oxygen levels greater than 50torr may cause oxygen toxicity.

Neonatal mechanical ventilation

The most obvious need for mechanical ventilation occurs when blood gases are unacceptable despite other methods of ventilatory support. It is important for the respiratory therapist to recognize and anticipate possible scenarios that frequently lead to the need for mechanical ventilation. The following list provides a brief summary:

- The most common is RDS
- Hypoventilation or apnea
- Severe disease or infection
- Prophylactic mechanical ventilation
- Aspiration of meconium
- Remember that oxygenation is improved in the neonate by using the following guideline:
- Oxygenation is dependent on mean airway pressure and fractional oxygen inspired.
- Use the lowest setting of FIO2 possible.
- In order to increase mean airway pressure, increase PIP, use PEEP up to 7cm H20, and increase inspiratory time up to 1.2seconds.

Ventilator parameters for neonates with PPH

Initial oxygen flows are 5-8L/min. PEEP should be avoided due to fragile pulmonary capillaries. Postductal Pa02 should be maintained >55torr. When high respiratory rates are needed, decrease inspiratory time from the normal. (.4-.7 seconds.) Remember that higher tidal volumes may be necessary to hyperventilate. Shunt studies determine the need for mechanical hyperventilation. Pre and post ductal blood sampling should be performed to diagnose shunting. Preductal and postductal oxygen levels should be the same. Echocardiogram is used to diagnose patent foramen ovale. Hyperventilation therapy is necessary for the neonate whose tests are positive for PPH. It is usually performed for 1-2 days. The goal of mechanical hyperventilation therapy is to reduce shunting. The neonate will be pharmacologically paralyzed to provide synchronized breathing. Small amounts of nitric oxide may be used for inhalation to dilate the pulmonary vessels. Special equipment is needed to measure and to deliver nitric oxide and the respiratory therapist should become familiar with the equipment.

Carbogen

Infants diagnosed with hypoplastic left heart syndrome (HLHS) do not have adequate circulation. Blood reaches the heart through patency of the ductus arteriosus (PDA). If the PDA closes before HLHS has been diagnosed, the infant develops respiratory distress. Until the condition is corrected, the ductus arteriosus must remain open. This is accomplished with intravenous medication, but the infant who is mechanically ventilated will receive Carbogen to constrict the pulmonary blood vessels and help maintain the PDA. The Carbogen is administered through a gas cylinder connected to the ventilator with a T-piece. Adjustments are made based on blood gas analysis. Carbogen administration requires close patient monitoring. A capnometer is used to measure the carbon dioxide delivery.   The proper amount of carbon dioxide is determined by performing a carbon dioxide response curve test.

Medications

Sedatives

Sedatives are needed when a patient is uncooperative and it becomes impossible to provide care.   Patients who have experienced head trauma become agitated as do patients who experience hypovolemia from blood loss. Confused states brought about by hypoxemia and brain disorders cause agitation. Patients with increased intracranial pressure must be sedated or paralyzed to decrease cerebral blood flow through mechanical hyperventilation. Many patients fight to extubate themselves. It's important to evaluate whether your patient is experiencing pain and should be given an analgesic such as Morphine. Commonly used sedatives are benzodiazepines such as Valium, Ativan, Xanax and Versed. Oversedation can be reversed with the drug Romazicon. Persons who are addicted to benzodiazepines can have seizures and become very combative after receiving Romazicon, Safety measures must be taken. Romazicon is used to "wake up" patients with benzodiazepine overdose. Sleeping medications are considered sedative-hypnotics because they assist with sleep. Barbituates produce a greater hypnotic effect that non barbituate hypnotics. Chloral Hydrate is a nonbarbituate and is safe for use in children or in elderly patients. Other examples include Nembutal, Pentothal, and Seconal.

Corticosteroid

Corticosteroids are used to treat many conditions, including lung disease. Corticosteroids are normally produced by the adrenal gland. When given in medication form, corticosteroids induce an adrenal effect. They reduce inflammation in the lungs. Corticosteroids also boost the effect of sympathomimetics. Corticosteroids can be given orally, intravenously, intranasal, or by inhalation. They have many side effects. When given by way of inhalation the side effects are minimized because there is little absorption into the systemic circulation. Intravenous corticosteroids are given in emergencies. Common examples of inhaled steroids are Advair Diskus, Vancenase, Azmacort and Flovent. Systemic examples (oral, I.V. or I.M.) include Deltasone, Solu Cortef, Prednisone, Prednisolone and Medrol. Systemic corticosteroids can cause adrenal insufficiency if stopped suddenly.

Vasoconstrictors

The patient who is receiving vasoconstrictors for a cardiac problem will be closely monitored for changes in both cardiac and pulmonary status. It's important for the respiratory therapist to understand the physiology of intravenous vasoconstrictors as it relates to the pulmonary vasculature and the expected results during use. Vasoconstrictors will cause peripheral circulation to diminish. This is an important factor when using pulse oximetry, because the decreased perfusion to the extremities will yield inaccurate results.

When measuring SVR, know that vasoconstrictors will increase SVR. Increased SVR can also be the result of fluid/volume overload, but it is important to know the patient's complete clinical status when making decisions regarding respiratory support. Normal SVR is 900-1400dynes/sec cm5 in the adult patient. When cardiac output is increased by the use of vasoconstrictors the PVR will also become elevated. Normal PVR is 80-240 dynes/sec cm5. You can see the importance of monitoring the cardiac and pulmonary status of the patient and how very frequent monitoring and adjustments to ventilation and drug administration become necessary.

Common emergency medications

Epinephrine is a vasoconstrictor. It is a first line medication used during CPR. It can be given intravenously or by endotracheal tube. Other vasoconstrictors may be added. Common examples are Levophed and Dopamine. Vasoconstrictors are used to raise blood pressure when it falls below levels that will perfuse the vital organs. Dopamine is often used to increase blood flow to the kidneys in low doses. Dopamine is a powerful vasoconstrictor when given in high doses. Antiarrhythmic drugs are given to treat bradycardia, tachycardia and ventricular tachycardia. Lidocaine is given for ventricular tachycardia and to reduce ventricular irritability after cardioversion or defibrillation. Atropine and epinephrine increase the heart rate and raise blood pressure. Inderal and Procainamide slow the heart rate. Nipride is used to lower blood pressure during a hypertensive crisis. Many drugs are available to control blood pressure and reduce the workload of the heart.

Remove Bronchopulmonary Secretions

Loosening secretions and promoting airway clearance

Patients need to be taught how to loosen secretions and promote airway clearance. Teach the patient to cough and deep breathe. Review patient exercises for muscle strengthening, and diaphragmatic breathing for debilitated patients. Medication or normal saline can be provided by way of aerosol to promote expectoration of sputum. Observe and document your findings regarding sputum production. Normal saline or sterile water helps liquefy secretions. Teach deep breathing and cough after the administration of aerosol solutions. Mucolytics, such a Mucomyst, can be used following an aerosol treatment with a bronchodilator. Mucomyst has a very noxious odor. The odor is consistently likened to that of rotten eggs. It can cause nausea. Mucomyst can have a bronchoconstrictive effect when used for asthma patients. It can be given by hand held nebulizer or with IPPB. Mucomyst can be placed directly into the trachea to loosen secretions. Proteolytic agents and mucolytics liquefy secretions. Dornase, or Pulmozyne is used to treat secretions by breaking up DNA strands. It is classified as a recombinant human deoxyribonuclease (RhDNAse) and is approved for use patients with lung infection complicated by cystic fibrosis.

Postural drainage therapy

Postural drainage is not ideal for critically ill patients because proper positioning is almost impossible. You must assess the benefit and only use this therapy when the results are certain to be positive for the patient. Gauge the patient's level of comfort and if the procedure causes pain stop the treatment. Reposition the patient, document the patient's response and communicate the any complaints to the physician. Vomiting can occur. If the patient should aspirate call for help provide oxygen. Clear the airway with suctioning. The patient's physician must be notified to evaluate the patient. If ineffective cough or bronchospasm occurs, stop therapy and provide oxygen. Recommend Mucolytics or aerosol to loosen secretions. Patients who have high blood pressure should be monitored closely. Stop treatment if the patient complains of headache or dizziness. If evidence of hypoxemia is present, reposition the patient and provide 100% oxygen. Notify the physician of any undesired outcomes.

Bronchopulmonary hygiene

It is the respiratory therapist's responsibility to teach and demonstrate cough and deep breathing. Feedback to the patient, from the therapist should be offered regularly, especially when the patient is weak or in pain. The COPD and surgical patient should understand that proper cough technique is part of disease management and stabilization. COPD patients who are weak or have thick secretions should be instructed to cough gently several times to raise secretions. A hard cough should be performed if the patient is capable. Show the patient how to loosen secretions by breathing through the nose several times followed by oral exhalation. Demonstrate by taking a deep breath, hold, and then exhale. Instruct the patient not to strain or take too large a breath. Have the patient sit upright to facilitate the use of large muscle groups. Preoperative teaching should be provided to patients to prevent atelectasis. After surgery, splint the patient's incision with a pillow to help with pain control and prevent wound dehiscence. The same breathing techniques discussed for overall pulmonary hygiene should be use for the postoperative patient.

Postural drainage to the upper lobes of the lungs

The patient should be positioned comfortably and safely; leaning slightly forward. The physician will provide specific orders regarding percussion and vibration. Once the patient is positioned properly, therapy is directed to the right, left, or both lungs by percussing and/or vibrating on either side of the spine. To provide therapy to the anterior lungs the patient is supine. Percussion or vibration is delivered to either or both sides, between the clavicle and the nipple area. Female are not likely to tolerate this type of procedure. The apical lung segment is treated as the patient leans backward and is performed between the scapula and clavicle. Postural drainage should be recommended when the patient's chest x-ray shows white shadows that could indicate atelectasis. Repeat the chest x-ray following therapy. Evaluate the patient's response and modify your treatment accordingly.

Respiratory therapy outcomes

Your patient must be able to tolerate the procedure you are providing. Oxygen should be humidified when patient comfort becomes an issue. Patients who use nasal cannulas can become sensitive to treatments. Inhalations can become uncomfortable. Dilute aerosols in the nebulizer with more saline or water when mucosal irritation is present. Decrease the amount for faster delivery when relief is needed quickly, such as during an asthma attack. Monitor the outcomes of each therapy and discuss with the doctor and nurses. Chart patient improvements or adverse treatment effects. Evaluate breath sounds and re-evaluate spirometry results. Observe changes in sputum production and cough. After coughing, listen again to the airways. Chart all patient outcomes, including self medication and remember that the goal is to prevent and treat recurrences of hospitalization. Treatments and recommendations are designed to help the patient remain as active as possible. Recommend changes in therapy as needed.

Maintain Airway

Airway protection

Position the patient to protect the airway. In an unconscious adult, the chin should be lifted and the head tilted to open the airway. Patients who are weak and debilitated must be positioned to prevent aspiration. Fowlers' or Semi-Fowler's position can be used. If the patient can't tolerate sitting up, they should be tilted slightly on their side and proper body alignment should be maintained. Make certain the mouth and nose are free from obstruction. A patient who has suffered stroke, trauma or surgery should have a properly fitted airway in place. If an oral airway cannot be used, the nasopharyngeal airway is indicated. Nasal intubation can be performed if trauma is present to the face, neck or jaw. During seizures or other conditions that could produce injury to the airway, an oropharyngeal airway is used to prevent biting. A laryngeal mask airway provides a means of ventilation without endotracheal intubation. Observe for aspiration when using any artificial airway. Never force an airway and be certain it is the correct size. Lubrication is used to prevent trauma.

Endotracheal intubation

When a patient's airway is compromised, endotracheal intubation is a safe, fast method to secure the airway. Sometimes the decision to intubate must be made very quickly. Use a tube that is the smallest cuff size and diameter to do the job. The smallest endotracheal tube has a diameter of 4mm; the largest is 14mm. The mean adult size used is 7-8mm. Nasal endotracheal tubes are slightly longer. The inner diameter of adult tubes varies with the length. Armored tubes are ideal for use because they prevent obstruction if the patient bites. The pediatric patient, under age eight should be intubated using a tube without a cuff. Nasal intubation is performed without a laryngoscope. It is easily accomplished because of a wire which is embedded in the tube. The wire serves as a guide into the trachea. Specialty tubes with more than one lumen can be used for jet ventilation. Special procedures, such as pneumonectomy and bronchoscopy require the use of a double lumen tube to ventilate one lung. An adaptor is available to ventilate both lungs.

It is possible to traumatize the mouth, teeth and vocal cords. Disturbances in heart rate and rhythm should be observed. Stomach contents, teeth and blood can be aspirated. Neck injury can occur if the neck is hyperextended. Prolonged intubation causes hoarseness. If too much cuff pressure is applied, injury and ischemia will result. Infection can occur. The tube can advance too far and end up in the right mainstem bronchus. Absence of breath sounds in the left lung; abdominal distention and lack of chest movement during manual ventilation indicate that the tube should be withdrawn 1-2cm. Esophageal intubation can cause gastric emptying and aspiration when the tube is removed. The patient can perform self extubation.   Routinely check for proper placement. Listen to breath sounds, note Chest X-ray results, use the exhaled CO_2 detector and check cuff pressure frequently (maintain at

15mmHg.) Cuff leaks can be heard over the larynx. Change the endotracheal tube if the cuff requires more than 20mmHg to seal an air leak.

<u>Endotracheal tube placement</u>

If you enter a patient's room, the ventilator is alarming, and you cannot hear breath sounds on the left side, withdraw the endotracheal tube 2-4 cm. and recheck breath sounds. Accidental endotracheal tube displacement occurs easily with patient movement and transport due to the flexibility of the tube. After the tube is repositioned and breath sounds are audible bilaterally, placement should be confirmed via chest X-Ray. Proper endotracheal tube placement by X-ray is confirmed when the tip is several centimeters below the vocal cords and several centimeters above the carina. The tube should be positioned mid trachea. Other assessment tools for proper endotracheal tube placement include assessment of breath sounds, observation of symmetrical chest movement bilaterally, auscultation of the abdomen for esophageal intubation, visualization by direct laryngoscopy and use of end tidal CO_2 monitor. Chest X-Ray is always needed for absolute verification.

SIMV mechanical ventilation

SIMV is synchronous mandatory ventilation. The patient is allowed to take breaths that are pressure supported. A preset rate delivers synchronized ventilation to the patient. Mandatory breaths are delivered at a set rate. In other words, the patient receives:

1. Synchronized breaths
2. Pressure supported breaths
3. Ventilator controlled breaths.

SIMV is used for patients who are breathing on their own. When using SIMV the patient's pressure waveform must be monitored to ensure correct inspiratory flow. As the patient begins to improve, pressure support can be decreased. If CO_2 levels rise, increase the respiratory rate. Tidal volume is set at 6ml/kg. but can be reduced if CO_2 levels rise. SIMV is most useful for patients who are breathing, but can't control the rate and length of inhalation and exhalation. SIMV is most often used during short term ventilatory support.

Controlled ventilation (C), assist control (AC) ventilation and pressure control ventilation (PCV)

Controlled ventilation is used for patients who have apnea. It is used when a patient needs to be medicinally paralyzed or heavily sedated. The use of control ventilation is otherwise limited because it does not allow the patient to breathe on his own. Assist control lets the patient take breaths from the ventilator while also receiving a preset delivered rate. The tidal volume that is delivered is consistent whether the machine delivers the breath or the patient initiates a breath. Pressure control ventilation is the same as assist control, with the exception that the tidal volumes vary. The tidal volume breaths are pressure limited and delivered in cycles. Because of the variations in tidal volume, the patient must be closely observed for respiratory failure.

Increased airway resistance

When managing increased airway resistance, evaluate the patient's WOB. Check airway resistance when the mechanically ventilated patient's breathing is desynchronized. Perform a pressure/volume loop then adjust the ventilator settings to decrease the patient's workload. Measure the pressure waveforms while the patient receives a ventilator delivered breath. The volume loop and waveform graphs should be compared to previous graphs. Look for evidence of air trapping. Exhaled volumes should return to baseline when graphed. Auto PEEP occurs when gas trapping increases and the I:E ratio increases. Use a pressure manometer to measure auto-PEEP while the patient is exhaling. Record the results as the total amount of PEEP. It may be necessary to increase therapeutic PEEP to match the total. The inspiratory time can also be decreased to allow for longer expiration. You may also wish to adjust the Tidal volume. Make changes and draw blood for analysis following each change. Take other measures to improve the expiratory time.

Check for bronchospasm and secretions. Airway resistance should be calculated after therapy has been adjusted.

Mechanical ventilation in the presence of ARDS

ARDS produces lung edema from fluid seeping into the alveoli. ARDS is the result of an underlying condition, it is a symptom and it can be life threatening. Oxygenation can be a challenge. Use of PCIRV prevents volutrauma from too large a tidal volume delivery and increases the inspiratory time. Tidal volume may be set as low as 6ml/kg. of body weight Keep the plateau pressure at 35cm.or less. Positive pressure ventilation is used to expand the alveoli. Lung compliance is low due to stiffness of the vascular bed. Oxygen shunting occurs, so it's important to perform studies. Constant volumes should be administered. If oxygen levels are low, adjust the inspiratory time to produce PCIRV. It takes longer for the fluid filled alveoli to fill.

Weaning parameters

The decision to wean a patient from mechanical ventilation depends on several factors. Several, but not all conditions should be present. The patient must be breathing spontaneously, with stable blood gas values. PaO2 level should be greater than 80 torr. Tidal volume should be 7-0ml/kg body weight. Vital signs should be stable. The patient's nutritional status should be optimal. PC02 should be at the patient's individual baseline or normal. Note overall patient improvement and correction of underlying disorders. Once weaning is started the patient must be closely monitored.

The endotracheal tube remains in place to protect the airway and provide a means for quick ventilatory support should the patient fail to wean. Initially, the respiratory therapist will observe the patient constantly, assessing the work of breathing, observing vital signs, and noting inspiratory, expiratory and tidal volumes. Sometimes the patient is removed from mechanical ventilation for increasingly longer periods until breathing is independent.

If a first weaning attempt fails, recommend gradual weaning. If the patient has been mechanically ventilated for a long period of time, use IMV/SIMV modes to wean.

Oropharyngeal airway insertion

An improperly inserted oral airway is of little benefit. Know the indications for use. The oropharyngeal airway should be used in an unconscious patient to protect the airway. The oropharyngeal airway prevents the tongue from obstructing the posterior pharynx. Use the correct size. Many practitioners accomplish oropharyngeal airway insertion by turning it upside down and gently rotating as it touches the soft palate. A tongue blade can be used to depress the tongue and insert the airway toward the back to the pharynx. If the patient is biting or seizing take precautions to avoid injury. It's possible to push the tongue back and cause further obstruction. Check the patient for loose teeth or dentures.

Nasopharyngeal airway insertion

Use a nasopharyngeal airway when the patient has an obstructed oral airway from trauma or surgery or when insertion of an oral airway is otherwise impossible. Choose the correct size. A t beveled tip airway is placed so that the opening is directed toward the septum. Blunt tip nasopharyngeal airways are available. Nasopharyngeal airways are also referred to as nasal trumpets. The nasopharyngeal airway can act as a guide for suctioning and can be used during bronchoscopy. The flexibility of this type of airway isn't as effective in keeping the tongue forward as is the harder oropharyngeal airway, but it can be less traumatic to mucosa when frequent suctioning is needed.

Airway suctioning

Airway suctioning is performed to remove secretions from the mouth and trachea. Weak and lethargic patients are unable to clear their own airways. Endotracheal and tracheostomy suctioning are sterile procedures. Suctioning through the nose and mouth are "clean" procedures. Hypoxemia, aspiration and vagal stimulation are possible during suctioning and should be avoided. The patient should be oxygenated with 100% 02 prior to the procedure. If the patient is already hypoxic limit the amount of time spent on the procedure. Increase FI02 first. Limit the amount of oxygen in infants due to the chance of retrolental fibroplasia. Use a non rebreathing mask for the patient who is breathing spontaneously. Deliver 100% oxygen to the patient on the ventilator, perform the procedure then reoxygenate. Stop if it is not tolerated. Use the lowest level of vacuum possible. Use sterile saline when needed to loosen secretions. Evaluate the patient before and after treatment.

Practice Test

Practice Questions

1. A patient comes to the emergency department with dyspnea and productive cough. Which of the following tests is NOT appropriate upon initial examination?
    a. Chest x-ray
    b. Pulse oximetry
    c. Arterial blood gas
    d. Vital sign assessment

2. Which of the following best describes a baby with a gestational age of 36 weeks?
    a. Term
    b. Preterm
    c. Not viable
    d. None of the above

3. A patient on mechanical ventilation has the following arterial blood gas results: pH of 7.35, CO_2 of 50 mmol/L, and HCO_3 of 24 mmol/L. Based on these results, how should this blood gas be classified?
    a. Respiratory alkalosis
    b. Respiratory acidosis
    c. Metabolic acidosis
    d. Within normal limits

4. Which of the following best describes the expected result of performing a complete pulmonary function test on a 60-year-old patient with chronic obstructive pulmonary disease?
    a. Normal lung volumes with limited expiratory flow
    b. Scooped-out flow volume loop
    c. All of the above
    d. None of the above

5. A 34-week-gestation infant is born via cesarean delivery. Despite stimulation, the patient is cyanotic and limp. Respirations are 10/min and heart rate is 72/min. Breath sounds are clear and diminished. Which of the following should be done first?
    a. Perform chest compressions.
    b. Ventilate the patient using a resuscitation bag and mask.
    c. Continue to stimulate the patient with rigorous rubbing of the body.
    d. Place the patient on a pulse oximetry monitor.

6. A patient comes to the emergency department with a productive cough, greenish sputum, and fever. The patient has had shortness of breath and coughing at night. The patient's temperature is 101.1 °F, respiratory rate is 22/min, heart rate is 110/min, and oxygen saturation is 92%. The physician performs percussion on this patient, and the notes are dull. Which of the following is the most likely diagnosis?
    a. Emphysema
    b. Pulmonary edema
    c. Pneumonia
    d. Status asthmaticus

7. A 30-year-old woman with chest discomfort is admitted to the hospital and is placed in the medical/surgical department. A physician is speaking with her for the first time. Which of the following pieces of information should the physician ask of the patient during this initial assessment?
    a. Past medical history
    b. Smoking history
    c. Current medications
    d. All of the above

8. A 75-year-old man with pneumonia appears confused and agitated. Which of the following questions should the physician ask to assess this patient's psychological state?
    a. "Can you tell me what day today is?"
    b. "Do you know where you are right now?"
    c. "What is your last name?"
    d. All of the above

9. A 47-year-old man, who has no pulse and is not breathing, is brought to the emergency department in an ambulance. Cardiopulmonary resuscitation is performed; the patient regains a pulse and is placed on mechanical ventilation. A chest x-ray is preformed post-intubation. The radiologist's report indicates: "Endotracheal tube is positioned 4 cm above the carina. Lung fields appear clear and equal with no infiltrates or effusions. Nasogastric tube appears to be in place." Which of the following statements is true regarding the above scenario?
    a. The endotracheal tube is in the proper position and needs no further assessment.
    b. The endotracheal tube is too large.
    c. The endotracheal tube is not in deep enough.
    d. The endotracheal tube position should be confirmed with an exhaled CO2 monitor.

10. A 2-year-old patient is brought to an urgent care facility with upper airway stridor, fever, and dyspnea. The patient appears sweaty and is drooling. A high-pitched barky cough is noted. Which of the following tests should be ordered for this patient?
    a. Chest x-ray
    b. Neck radiograph
    c. Pulse oximetry
    d. All of the above

11. A 2-year-old patient is brought to an urgent care facility with upper airway stridor, fever, and dyspnea. The patient appears sweaty and is drooling. A high-pitched barky cough is noted. A neck radiograph is completed, which shows a column of air around the epiglottis. A physician says that he sees the "thumb sign." What is the most likely diagnosis?
    a. Croup
    b. Epiglottitis
    c. Asthma
    d. Allergic reaction

12. A patient with an oxygen saturation of 88%, a heart rate of 75/min, and an irregular pulse oximeter waveform says that she is cold. Which of the following actions is NOT appropriate at this time?
    a. Take the patient's pulse.
    b. Inspect the patient's hands.
    c. Change the sensor.
    d. Place the patient on a 2-L nasal cannula.

13. A patient is diaphoretic and anxious, has chest pain, and feels dizzy and "jittery." The physician checks her electrocardiogram (EKG) strip and sees a narrow QRS complex and a heart rate of 180/min. What is the most likely diagnosis?
    a. Supraventricular tachycardia
    b. Sinus tachycardia
    c. Ventricular fibrillation
    d. Ventricular tachycardia

14. A patient is diaphoretic and anxious, has chest pain, and feels dizzy and "jittery." The physician checks her electrocardiogram (EKG) strip and sees a narrow QRS complex and a heart rate of 180/min. Which of the following is the most appropriate FIRST treatment plan?
    a. Defibrillation
    b. Cardioversion
    c. Adenosine
    d. Vagal maneuvers

15. A 150-kg patient is admitted for bariatric surgery. Heart rate is 70/min, oxygen saturation is 87%, and the waveform is regular. The patient is snoring loudly. The physician is called, and he gives a telephone order to start the patient on bilevel positive airway pressure. What settings are appropriate for this patient, including inspiratory positive airway pressure (IPAP), expiratory positive airway pressure (EPAP), fraction of inspired oxygen (FiO_2), and continuous positive airway pressure (CPAP)?
    a. IPAP 10, EPAP 5, FiO2 21%
    b. IPAP 5, EPAP 10, FiO2 30%
    c. IPAP 10, EPAP 5, FiO2 30%
    d. CPAP 5, FiO2 21%

16. A physician is called to provide asthma education for the mother of a pediatric patient. The patient is allergic to dogs and cats, and the family owns one dog. The patient's father smokes in the home, and the mother is a former smoker. How should the physician educate the parents on trigger avoidance in the home?
    a. Encourage the father to stop smoking in the home and car.
    b. Tell the mother to tell her husband to quit smoking.
    c. Explain that the dog can sleep in the patient's bedroom as long as it is not near the patient's pillow.
    d. Encourage the parents to replace the dog with a hypoallergenic dog.

17. A patient in the adult intensive care unit is on mechanical volume ventilation. The vent is alarming "high airway pressure." The patient has a heart rate of 110/min and a blood pressure of 80/50 mm Hg, and is desaturating. Upon auscultation, the physician hears diminished breath sounds on the right, with clear breath sounds on the left. A portable chest x-ray shows left tracheal deviation and mediastinum shift. The patient has an increased percussion note. Which of the following respiratory disorders is most consistent with these symptoms?
    a. Left tension pneumothorax
    b. Right tension pneumothorax
    c. Left traumatic pneumothorax
    d. Right traumatic pneumothorax

18. Which of the following best describes the optimal peak flow technique?
    a. The patient stands, takes the biggest breath they can, and blows it out hard and fast through the peak flow meter. Repeat 2 more times and report the highest number.
    b. The patient stands, takes the biggest breath they can, and blows it out hard and fast through the peak flow meter. Repeat 3 more times and report the average number.
    c. The patient sits up straight, takes the biggest breath they can, and blows it out hard and fast through the peak flow meter. Repeat 3 more times and report the average number.
    d. The patient stands, takes the biggest breath they can, and blows it out hard and fast through the peak flow meter. Repeat 1 more time and report the highest number.

19. A the patient performs the peak flow technique correctly, and reaches a number of 150. The patient's predicted peak flow is 310. The patient is in what peak flow zone at this time?
    a. Yellow zone
    b. Green zone
    c. Red zone
    d. None of the above

20. A patient in the intensive care unit is on mechanical ventilation, and the physician wants to know whether or not the patient has auto peep. Which of the following choices best describes what auto peep looks like on the ventilator graphics screen?

a. On the flow-time curve, expiratory flow does not return to zero before inhalation begins.

b. On the flow-time curve, expiratory flow returns to zero before inhalation begins.

c. One cannot determine if the patient has auto peep from the ventilator graphics.

d. None of the above describes the appearance of auto peep on a ventilator graphics screen.

21. A patient is on the following vent settings: assist control, tidal volume 500, rate 14, PEEP of 7, and 35% FIO2. An arterial blood gas is drawn, and the patient's Pa CO_2 is 80 and PaO2 is 75. Barometric pressure is 29.95 inches of Hg. What is the patient's PAO2?

a. -105.97

b. 100

c. 75

d. 149.81

22. A patient is on the following vent settings: assist control, tidal volume 500, rate 14, PEEP of 7, and 35% FIO2. An arterial blood gas is drawn, and the patient's Pa CO_2 is 80 and PaO2 is 75. Barometric pressure is 29.95 inches of Hg. What is this patient's A-a gradient?

a. 69.81

b. -185.97

c. 20

d. 5

23. During electrocardiogram (EKG), a patient experiences chest tightness and anxiety. The patient is restless and says he "can't get comfortable." The EKG printout shows a rhythm that appears to be ventricular tachycardia. The patient is still speaking and is in no distress. Pulse is 80/min. What of the following is the best interpretation of this rhythm?

a. The patient is in ventricular tachycardia and must be treated immediately.

b. The patient's movement and agitation may have caused artifact on the EKG rhythm strip, and further evaluation is required.

c. The patient is having a heart attack.

d. None of the above is accurate.

24. Which of the following statements is or are true of pseudomonas?

a. It is a gram-negative bacterium.

b. It is an aerobic bacterium.

c. It is characterized by sweet-smelling sputum.

d. All of the above are true.

25. A patient is admitted on the general medical floor of a hospital with an admitting diagnosis of congestive heart failure. His breath sounds are diminished on auscultation and he has a dull percussion note. Which of the following tests might be helpful in diagnosis?
    a. Chest CT scan
    b. Chest x-ray
    c. Ultrasound
    d. All of the above

26. Which of the following actions can be performed via bronchoscope?
    a. Visual inspection of the airways
    b. Removal of foreign body or tissue
    c. Airway clearance
    d. All of the above

27. Which of the following is true of the laryngeal mask airway?
    a. It is a mask that fits over the nose and mouth and assists in ventilation with ambu bag.
    b. It is most commonly used in surgery and emergency situations.
    c. It is not an effective way to ventilate a patient.
    d. None of the above is true.

28. A 49-year-old man, weighing 133 kg, has just had bariatric surgery. He has a history of claustrophobia and is nervous about using a continuous positive airway pressure (CPAP) machine. Which of the following is the most appropriate advice regarding the selection of a CPAP mask for this patient?
    a. Choose a full-face mask because that's what most patients require.
    b. Choose a nasal mask size based on the patient's body-mass index (BMI).
    c. Tell the patient he can't successfully use a CPAP machine if he has claustrophobia.
    d. None of the above is appropriate.

29. A 49-year-old man, weighing 133 kg, has just had bariatric surgery. He has a history of claustrophobia and is nervous about using a continuous positive airway pressure (CPAP) machine. Which of the following methods will best help to make this patient's CPAP treatment more tolerable?
    a. Choose a mask of the appropriate size and shape.
    b. Set a ramp setting on the patient's machine, if available.
    c. Choose a mask of the appropriate size and shape and set a ramp setting on his machine.
    d. Tell the patient to calm down.

30. A baby is on pressure control ventilation with the following settings: PIP 20, peep 5, 26% FIO2, rate 30. Which of the following is true about this patient's ventilator settings?
    a. Total pressure is 20.
    b. Total pressure is 15 .
    c. Pressure control ventilation is volume limited.
    d. Pressure control is a spontaneous mode.

31. A 75-year-old man with a history of chronic obstructive pulmonary disease (COPD) is receiving in-home respiratory care. He states that his portable oxygen concentrator is not giving him enough flow. Which of the following is NOT an appropriate way to troubleshoot his equipment?
    a. Check the tubing for kinks, holes, leaks, or other damage.
    b. Add an extension to the patient's tubing and then check the flow.
    c. Check the humidifier for cracks or loose connections.
    d. All of the above options are appropriate.

32. Which of the following statements is true regarding quality control on blood gas analyzers in the intensive care unit?
    a. The medical director does not need to oversee the quality control measures.
    b. Quality control measures should be performed a minimum of every 12 hours.
    c. Quality control policy should not include remediation protocols.
    d. None of the above is true.

33. A 14-year-old boy with a chronic cough is undergoing a complete pulmonary function test. The following baseline information is collected: FVC 95%, FEV1 75%, FEF25-75 77%, TLC 114%, VC 97%, FRC 136%, RV 135%. He then receives a handheld nebulizer treatment of 2.5 mg albuterol and tests are repeated. The following information is collected: FVC 95%, FEV1 90%, FEF25-75 89%, TLC 114%, VC 97%, FRC135%, RV 138%. This test shows that the patient
    a. has a restrictive disease.
    b. has asthma.
    c. has an obstructive lung disorder.
    d. gave poor effort.

34. When treating a patient with a history of clostridium difficile, which of the following pieces of protective equipment is or are required to prevent the spread of this disease within the unit?
    a. Gloves
    b. Gown
    c. Mask
    d. Gloves and gown

35. If an avian flu pandemic were to break out, which of the following steps to contain and prevent the spread of the illness is or are most appropriate?
a. Encourage all health care workers to exercise good hand hygiene.
b. Require all health care workers to wear personal protective equipment including a respirator mask, gown, and gloves.
c. Place patients in airborne isolation.
d. All of the above steps should be taken.

36. A patient with a history of chronic obstructive pulmonary disease (COPD) is admitted for pneumonia. Nebulizer treatments with 2.5 mg of albuterol have been ordered every four hours and as needed for wheezing. Before treatment, the patient's respiratory rate is 18/min, heart rate is 89/min, and breath sounds are diminished in all lobes. After treatment, the patient's respiratory rate is 19/min, heart rate is 95/min, and breath sounds include inspiratory and expiratory wheezing. The patient is now coughing up small amounts of yellow sputum. Which of the following statements regarding the patient's condition is true?
a. The patient is experiencing an adverse reaction to the treatment and the doctor must be notified.
b. The treatment has improved the patient's condition.
c. The treatment has made the patient worse, and should be discontinued.
d. The patient is in respiratory distress and should be given another treatment immediately.

37. A patient with a history of chronic obstructive pulmonary disease (COPD) is admitted for pneumonia. Nebulizer treatments with 2.5 mg of albuterol have been ordered every four hours and as needed for wheezing. Which of the following would indicate that this patient's treatment has had a positive outcome?
a. The patient experiences improved breath sounds, sputum clearance, and work of breathing.
b. Therapy is adjusted in accordance with the patient's goals for therapy.
c. The patient is no longer taking any respiratory medications, including daily inhalers.
d. Both A and B are achieved.

38. Which of the following are risk factors for ventilator-associated pneumonia?
a. Extended length of time on ventilator, supine patient position, condensation in ventilator circuit, and breaking of ventilator circuit
b. Semi-recumbent patient position, gastric reflux, and breaking of ventilator circuit
c. Shortened length of time on ventilator, semi-recumbent patient position, and gastric reflux
d. None of the above

39. Which of the following items is needed at the bedside in order to properly extubate a patient?
   a. Suction
   b. 10 cc syringe
   c. Supplemental oxygen
   d. All of the above

40. Which of the following is the correct sequence of events in performing an extubation?
   a. Suction the patient's endotracheal tube, deflate the cuff, ask the patient to take a deep breath in and blow it out while removing the tube, and place the patient on room air.
   b. Deflate the cuff, suction the patient's mouth and endotracheal tube, ask the patient to take a deep breath in and blow it out while removing the tube, and place the patient on supplemental oxygen as needed.
   c. Suction the patient's mouth and endotracheal tube, deflate the cuff, ask the patient to take a deep breath in and blow it out while removing the tube, and place patient on supplemental oxygen as needed.
   d. Suction the patient's endotracheal tube, deflate the cuff, ask the patient to take a deep breath in and blow it out while removing the tube, and place the patient on a nebulizer treatment of albuterol, 2.5 mg.

41. One disadvantage of inhaled corticosteroids is that they
   a. have severe adverse effects and should only be taken for short periods of time.
   b. hinder the activation of inflammatory cells in the lungs.
   c. are ineffective in controlling asthma symptoms.
   d. are not safe for use during pregnancy.

42. Which of the following choices best describes the proper technique for nasotracheal suctioning of a child?
   a. Using a measured suction and sterile technique, lubricate catheter using lubricating jelly, insert catheter into the patient's nare, and apply suction upon removal. Rinse catheter with sterile water or saline and repeat in 30-second intervals as tolerated. Discard catheter and kit after use.
   b. Wear examination gloves while inserting catheter into the patient's nare. Apply suction upon removal and rinse catheter with sterile water or saline. Repeat in 30-second intervals as tolerated.
   c. Keep used catheter and kit at patient's bedside for later use.
   d. Perform both B and C.

43. A 2-year-old boy is brought to the emergency department with tracheal tugging. Upon auscultation of the neck and chest, upper airway stridor and clear lung sounds are heard. The patient's oxygen saturation on room air is 96%. The mother states that the boy awakened in the middle of the night with a barking cough and hoarse voice. Which of the following nebulizer treatments is the best choice?
a. Albuterol, 2.5 mg
b. Ipratropium, 0.5 mg
c. Racemic epinephrine, 0.5 mL of 2.25%, plus 3 mL normal saline
d. None of the above

44. A 14-year-old patient with asthma is brought to the pediatric floor as a direct admission from the doctor's office. Heart rate is 110/min, respiratory rate is 25/min, and mild intercostal retractions are noted. A faint expiratory wheeze is noted upon auscultation. SPO2 is 90%. The patient has no prior history of breathing problems. He states he was playing football and became "winded" and started to cough. He says, "My chest feels tight." A portable chest x-ray is taken at the bedside and the results indicate that no active disease is present. The patient is speaking in full sentences. What is an appropriate course of treatment for this patient?
a. Provide asthma education and tell the patient that he must not participate in sports because it is exacerbating his asthma.
b. Give a 2.5 mg albuterol nebulizer treatment immediately, and give supplemental oxygen as needed.
c. Monitor the patient, give a 2.5 mg albuterol nebulizer treatment in one hour, and give supplemental oxygen as needed.
d. All of the above are appropriate treatments.

45. A 42-year-old patient has been using a fluticasone and salmeterol 500/50 inhaler daily for 2 weeks and has not felt any better yet. He also reports a sweet taste in his mouth after taking the medication. Which of the following actions is most appropriate in this situation?
a. Explain that this medication takes up to several weeks to work, and that the sweet taste is a normal side effect.
b. Change the patient to another medication, because this one is not working for him.
c. Tell the patient to use a spacer with this medication and instruct him on how to use it.
d. Perform both B and C.

46. Which of the following best describes the proper technique for performing an arterial blood gas?

    a. Ask the patient's name, place the patient's wrist on a rolled-up towel, perform an Allen test, clean the area with alcohol, insert the needle at a 45-degree angle with the bevel up and the head of the needle facing toward the patient, remove the needle when the syringe is full, put pressure on the puncture site, and cover with a bandage.

    b. Ask the patient's name, place the patient's wrist flat on the bed, perform an Allen test, clean the area with alcohol, insert the needle at a 45-degree angle with the bevel up and the head of the needled facing toward the patient, remove the needle when the syringe has an adequate sample, put pressure on the puncture site, and cover with a bandage.

    c. Identify the patient using 2 forms of identification, place the patient's wrist on a rolled-up towel, perform an Allen test, clean the area with alcohol, insert the needle at a 45-degree angle with the bevel up and the head of the needled going toward the patient, remove the needle when the syringe has an adequate sample, put pressure on the puncture site, and cover with a bandage.

    d. Identify the patient using 2 forms of identification, place the patient's wrist on a rolled-up towel, clean the area with alcohol, insert the needle at a 45-degree angle with the bevel up and the head of the needled going toward the patient, remove the needle when the syringe has an adequate sample, put pressure on the puncture site, and cover with a bandage.

47. Which of the following is or are true about capnography in adult patients?

    a. Capnography measures dead space and exhaled CO2.

    b. Capnography is noninvasive.

    c. Capnography can also be provided to neonatal and pediatric patients.

    d. All of the above are true.

48. A patient is on a Puritan Bennett 840 ventilator with the following settings: assist control, rate 18, TV 500, FI02 50%, +5 peep. The patient was placed on an end tidal CO_2 monitor last evening. During the last vent check, the patient's end tidal CO_2 monitor showed an even waveform with uniform waves. Then the CO_2 waveform becomes flattened to a straight line and the patient's ventilator starts alarming. What is the most likely explanation for this problem?

    a. The patient has become disconnected.

    b. The patient is hyperventilating.

    c. The patient has self-extubated.

    d. Both A and C have happened.

49. A 14-year-old girl with suspected asthma is receiving a methacholine challenge. She has shortness of breath with exercise and exposure to dogs and nighttime coughing and wheezing. Her primary physician suspects asthma; however, she had a pulmonary function test one month ago with normal results. The test did not show any percent change after administration of a bronchodilator, and the patient had normal volumes and flows on that test. Today she arrives at a pulmonary lab for a bronchoprovocation test. What is the best way to prepare this patient for the test?

    a. Do not warn her of possible bronchospasm from the methacholine because this may produce false values in the test.

    b. Explain to her that she may feel short of breath or wheeze during the test, but additional medication will reverse this effect.

    c. Tell her how long the test should take, what it will measure, and what is required of her during the test.

    d. Perform both B and C.

50. A 14-year-old girl has completed a methacholine challenge. On her pulmonary function test from last month, her FEV1 was 91%. During her bronchoprovocation challenge today, her FEV1 is 69%. What does this change in FEV1 indicate?

    a. The FEV1 is still within normal limits.

    b. The FEV1 drop shows a positive test result.

    c. This patient's diagnosis of asthma can be confirmed.

    d. Both B and C are true.

51. A patient in the adult intensive care unit has been resting comfortably all day. During ventilation, however, the patient grimaces and uses accessory muscles. The patient becomes sweaty and the ventilator alarms "high pressure." What is the most appropriate next step?

    a. Remove the patient from the ventilator and manually ventilate with 100% oxygen via ambu bag and mask.

    b. Check the patient for signs of endotracheal tube blockage, kinks in the tube, or other obstructions.

    c. Perform both A and B.

    d. Increase the high-pressure limit.

52. A man was admitted to the intensive care unit for respiratory failure. He is 5'7" and weighs 250 lbs. His vent settings are as follows: assist control, 900, 14, +5, 30%. His arterial blood gas results are: 7.45, 30, 90, 24. Based on this information, what ventilator setting should be changed?

    a. Tidal volume

    b. Rate

    c. Mode

    d. A and B

53. A 72-year-old man is in a motor vehicle accident. He is in the intensive care unit on a Puritan Bennett 840 ventilator. The patient settings are as follows: assist control, 500, 12, +5, 60%. Based on this information, which of the following information is needed to determine this patient's ability to be weaned from the ventilator?
    a. Negative inspiratory force
    b. Vital capacity
    c. Rapid shallow breathing index
    d. All of the above

54. A 34-year-old man was found unresponsive in his hospital room. He is 6'2" and weighs 247 lbs. The patient has no known pulmonary history. The doctor intubates with a size 7 endotracheal tube. After bagging, the CO_2 detector placed on the tube changes from purple to yellow. A gurgling sound comes from the patient's throat. After deflating and reinflating the cuff, a leak is still heard. What should be done next?
    a. Bag harder and faster to compensate for the leak.
    b. Recommend extubation and reintubate with a larger tube.
    c. Continue bagging. The leak will improve once the patient is placed on a ventilator.
    d. Push 10 more cc's of air into the patient's cuff to decrease the leak around the cuff.

55. A 12-year-old girl with a history of asthma and allergies is receiving home care. She experiences dyspnea and gasping while sleeping. She sleeps with one pillow and says that she feels like she is going to suffocate in the night. She says that she also has this problem during her yoga class when she has to lie on her back on the mat. To alleviate this patient's dyspnea, she should be told
    a. to sleep elevated.
    b. to take a cough suppressant at night.
    c. that this is a normal part of asthma and there is nothing that can be done.
    d. to use her inhaler during the night.

56. A patient in the adult intensive care unit is experiencing auto peep. His auto peep level is 7. Which of the following options is or are appropriate ways to lower and eliminate auto peep?
    a. Change the set peep level to 7.
    b. Lower the set frequency.
    c. Lower the set tidal volume.
    d. Perform all of the above.

57. A 68-year-old man is admitted for pneumonia. He is currently on 4 L/min of oxygen via nasal cannula. He experiences shortness of breath and cough at rest. He is coughing up small amounts of thick, yellow sputum. He states he feels congested but "can't cough it all out." Breath sounds are coarse with rhonchi and faint inspiratory wheezes. He exhibits increased accessory muscle use while resting. The patient is currently taking nebulizer treatments with albuterol and ipratropium, and acetylcysteine every 4 hours. Which of the following suggestions will help alleviate this patient's symptoms?
    a. Decrease nebulizer treatments and increase oxygen flow rate.
    b. Order positive expiratory pressure (PEP) therapy with each nebulizer treatment.
    c. Order nasotracheal suctioning as needed.
    d. None of the above will alleviate this patient's symptoms.

58. A 154-lb man in the adult intensive care unit has been on the ventilator for 10 days. The doctor wants to see if the patient is able to be weaned from the ventilator. Weaning parameters are performed on the patient with these results: vital capacity (VC) 4.9, negative inspiratory force (NIF) -23, rapid shallow breathing index (RSBI) 95. The patient is hemodynamically stable, alert, and resting comfortably. Given this information, which of the following statements is true?
    a. The patient's VC is low for his ideal bodyweight and therefore he is not ready to be weaned.
    b. The patient's NIF, VC, and RSBI are adequate and the weaning process can begin.
    c. The patient has been on the ventilator too long to be weaned at this time.
    d. None of the above is true.

59. When ventilating a patient with volume control ventilation, which of the following ventilator setting adjustments would decrease a patient's plateau pressures?
    a. Decreased tidal volume
    b. Increased tidal volume
    c. Increased FIO2
    d. None of the above

60. A 76-year-old woman is admitted for congestive heart failure. She has a history of lung cancer and cerebrovascular accident and is confused and sleepy. The patient's weight is 110 lbs. and her urine output today has been 15 mL/hour. Upon auscultation, the patient's breath sounds are coarse and wet with rales in all lobes. No wheezing is noted. The patient is receiving 2.5 mg albuterol nebulizer treatments every four hours. There is no change in the patient's status post nebulizer. Which of the following treatment choices would be the best recommendation at this time?
    a. Administer another nebulizer treatment.
    b. Give 20 mg furosemide.
    c. Start CPT with nebs.
    d. Perform both A and B.

61. A 28-week neonate is pink, with a heart rate of 110/mind and a respiratory rate of 35/min. The baby is grunting and exhibits intercostal and subcostal retractions. Which of the following choices would best help to reduce the incidence of respiratory distress syndrome in this patient?
    a. Intubate and administer surfactant.
    b. Place the patient on nasal prong CPAP.
    c. Manually ventilate the baby with ambu bag and mask.
    d. Perform both A and B.

62. Hospital protocol dictates that all qualifying patients must be offered a seasonal influenza shot during their admission. Which of the following patient populations would qualify for a flu shot according to the Centers for Disease Control and Prevention's (CDC's) current recommendations?
    a. A 7-month-old girl admitted with a diagnosis of failure to thrive
    b. A 16-year-old girl with asthma
    c. A 72-year-old man admitted for a hip fracture
    d. All of the above

63. Which of the following statements is true regarding the pneumococcal conjugate vaccine?
    a. Babies less than 12 months old should not take it.
    b. Adults with cold symptoms should not take it.
    c. Babies with fevers can take it.
    d. None of the above is true.

64. The emergency department director is working on forming a respiratory protocol for asthma patients in the emergency department. Which of the following criteria would be most appropriate to measure in the newly designed protocol?
    a. Breath sounds pre- and post-treatment and chest x-ray, if available
    b. Oxygen saturation, cough, and past medical history
    c. Pre- and post-peak-flow measurements, including personal best and predicted peak flows
    d. All of the above

65. A 16-year-old girl with cystic fibrosis was just admitted to the pediatric floor 1 hour ago. She has a history of asthma and seasonal allergies. The patient's breath sounds are slightly coarse and diminished. She states she feels well and is not having any trouble breathing. What other information is needed to determine which pharmacological therapy to order?
    a. Drug allergies, home medications, and when her last dose was given
    b. Food allergies
    c. Patient's normal activity level at home
    d. Both A and B

66. A 16-year-old girl with cystic fibrosis was just admitted to the pediatric floor 1 hour ago. She has a history of asthma and seasonal allergies. The patient's breath sounds are slightly coarse and diminished. She states she feels well and is not having any trouble breathing. She is discovered to be allergic to dairy products. The physician states that he would like to order fluticasone and salmeterol 250/50 for this patient due to her history of asthma. What is the most appropriate next step?

    a. Order the fluticasone and salmeterol diskus per the physician's request.
    b. Change the patient to fluticasone and salmeterol HFA 115mcg/21mcg with spacer.
    c. Change the patient to fluticasone and salmeterol HFA 230mcg/21mcg with spacer.
    d. Do not order fluticasone and salmeterol in any form.

67. A pediatric patient in the emergency department is being admitted for respiratory syncytial virus. The patient is a 2-year-old girl with a history of cough, wheezing, and fever for 3 days. The patient was given a home nebulizer by her doctor, and has been using 2.5 mg albuterol nebulizer treatments, every 4 hours and as needed. The patient was brought to the emergency department by ambulance and was given two 2.5 mg albuterol nebulizer treatments back to back in the ambulance. Upon auscultation, clear breath sounds with good aeration throughout can be heard. The patient's room air oxygen saturation is 95%. Which of the following orders is most appropriate for this patient?

    a. Monitor the patient for the next several hours and reassess later that day.
    b. Order nebulizer treatments with budesonide, 0.5 mg as needed, for wheezing.
    c. Order 2.5 mg nebulizer treatments every three hours and as needed for wheezing.
    d. Order CPT every 4 hours.

68. A 6-year-old boy has been in the hospital for over 5 days due to bronchitis. The doctor orders budesonide DPI, 1 puff twice daily, and 2 puffs albuterol metered dose inhaler with spacer as needed for wheezing. After the treatment plan is explained to her, the mother says, "I will not allow him to take steroids. They will stunt his growth and he will become addicted to them like those bodybuilders on TV." Which of the following options is the best choice for this situation?

    a. Tell the mother that budesonide is not the same as the anabolic steroids used for bodybuilding.
    b. Tell the mother that all medications have side effects but he will just have to live with them.
    c. Explain to the mother that while oral steroids have potentially serious side effects, the inhaled variety is very safe and effective for young children.
    d. Perform both A and C.

69. The mother in question 68 is still not comfortable with the patient using inhaled steroids. She says, "I don't understand why he needs that medicine. The albuterol works for him so why would I need another medication too? That's too much medicine for one little boy." What is the best thing to do in this situation?

    a. Discontinue the budesonide and increase the frequency of the albuterol to 4 puffs as needed.

    b. Educate the mother on the difference between controller and rescue medications and their role in the patient's medication regimen.

    c. Tell the doctor that the mother has refused the medication, and make a note in the patient's chart.

    d. Perform both A and C.

70. Rapid sequence intubation is being performed on a 75-kg patient admitted for drug overdose. The patient is restless, combative, and coughing. Which of the following is the best choice for this patient?

    a. Give propofol, 150 mg, followed by succinylcholine, 115 mg, then intubate.

    b. Give succinylcholine, 115 mg, then intubate.

    c. This patient can't be intubated due to his combativeness.

    d. No drugs are needed to intubate this patient.

71. When performing single-rescuer CPR on an adult, which of the following choices is the correct compression-to-breath ratio?

    a. 15:1

    b. 30:2

    c. 15:2

    d. 30:1

72. When in the CPR sequence should an AED be used?

    a. Immediately

    b. After 1 round of CPR

    c. After 2 rounds of CPR

    d. After 5 minutes of CPR

73. A critical status 29-week-gestation baby must be transported to a level 3 neonatal intensive care unit 110 miles away. The baby is on pressure control mechanical ventilation and is stable at this time. Which of the following are disadvantages to transporting this patient by helicopter?

    a. Altitude-related pressure changes

    b. Increased vibration and noise

    c. Small patient care area on board the aircraft

    d. All of the above

74. A 22-year-old man in the adult intensive care unit was admitted for chest pain. He is 6'3" and weighs 180 lbs. The patient states he was sitting in class when he had sudden onset of left-sided chest pain and shortness of breath. An electrocardiogram (EKG) was performed, and the results showed normal sinus tachycardia with a heart rate of 115/min. The patient experiences severe chest pain and the nurse administers morphine per the physician's order. A chest x-ray is taken, and on the film that the patient's left lung looks dark and the mediastinum has shifted to the right. Which of the following is the most likely diagnosis?

    a. Spontaneous primary pneumothorax
    b. Spontaneous secondary pneumothorax
    c. Left hemothorax
    d. Spontaneous Iatrogenic pneumothorax

75. You are asked to assist a physician in the placement of a chest tube on the patient in question 74. In what location is a chest tube normally placed for the treatment of a spontaneous pneumothorax in adults?

    a. Fourth or fifth intercostal space anterior in the anterior axillary line
    b. Sixth intercostal space in the mid clavicular line
    c. Third intercostal space in the mid clavicular line
    d. Second intercostal space in the anterior axillary line

76. What is the role of a registered respiratory therapist in assisting a pulmonologist with a thoracentesis?

    a. Monitoring the patient
    b. Providing supplemental oxygen as needed
    c. Inserting the needle and withdrawing fluid
    d. Both A and B

77. A patient in the pediatric intensive care unit will be going home later today. The patient's mother states that their home nebulizer is no longer working. She says she is afraid a new one won't be covered by insurance. Which of the following choices is the best action to take first in this situation?

    a. Tell the patient's mother that she will have to pay for a new nebulizer because the doctor wants the patient to take treatments at home.
    b. Change the patient's therapy to metered dose inhaler with spacer instead of nebulizer treatments.
    c. Talk to the patient's case manager about the broken nebulizer and follow up with the patient's mother.
    d. Take some nebulizer parts from the respiratory care equipment room and see if it will fix the problem.

78. A 13-year-old girl is admitted for cough and shortness of breath. She has a history of intermittent cough for 1 year. The cough is nonproductive and is worse with exercise and at night. The patient is afebrile and her breath sounds are clear in all lobes. The patient has been on antibiotics and prednisone intermittently for the past year. Which of the following tests would be helpful in making a diagnosis?
    a. Complete pulmonary function test
    b. Sleep study
    c. Arterial blood gas
    d. All of the above

79. A 65-year-old patient weighs 270 lbs. and is 5'8". He reports headache and daytime sleepiness. His wife states that she moved into the guest bedroom due to his constant snoring. The patient's blood pressure is 150/90 mm Hg and his oxygen saturation is 99%. Which of the following tests should be recommended for this patient?
    a. Continuous pulse oximetry monitoring during the day
    b. Sleep study
    c. Arterial blood gas
    d. Both B and C

80. A 76-year-old woman is being ventilated with noninvasive positive pressure ventilation via the Phillips Respironics Vision bilevel positive airway pressure (bipap). The patient is on spontaneous timed mode with a rate of 12, inspiratory positive airway pressure (Ipap) of 10, and expiratory positive airway pressure (Epap) of 5. The patient is wearing a full-face mask, and her FIO2 is 35%. The bipap is alarming low pressure and apnea. What should be done next?
    a. Turn the alarm limit up, as this is a nuisance alarm.
    b. Evaluate the patient for leaks in the system.
    c. Call for help and begin rescue breathing via ambu bag and mask.
    d. Perform both A and B.

81. A 21-year-old man is transported to the emergency department via ambulance. The patient was in a motor vehicle accident and was ejected from the car. The patient arrives at the emergency department with profuse bleeding in and around the airway, and extensive trauma to the face, nose, and chest. The physician attempts to orally intubate 3 times, but is unable to visualize the chords and the patient is starting to desaturate. Anesthesia is paged; however, a fiber-optic scope is not available at this time. What is the best suggestion in this situation?
    a. Use an esophageal tracheal combitube.
    b. Attempt nasal intubation.
    c. Reattempt oral intubation.
    d. Attempt noninvasive ventilation via bipap.

82. A patient has just been placed on a high-frequency oscillator. Her chest wiggle is from her neck to her waist. Which of the following statements is true regarding this patient?
a. No further action is required at this time.
b. The amplitude should be increased.
c. The amplitude should be decreased.
d. The mean pressure should be decreased.

83. Which of the following tests is or are included in the standardized daily quality control measures for pulmonary function equipment?
a. Volume
b. Time
c. Flow
d. Flow and volume

84. An 8-year-old boy's asthma diary shows the following peak flow measurements for this week: Sunday 310, Monday 300, Tuesday 450, Wednesday 100, Thursday 180, Friday 245, Saturday 330. Which of the following actions should be done next?
a. Evaluate the patient's peak flow technique.
b. Report the patient's Tuesday value of 450 as his personal best.
c. Ask the patient what his symptoms were on each of these days.
d. Perform both A and C.

85. While intubating a patient using an esophageal tracheal combitube, which of the following patient positions is most beneficial during the insertion of the combitube?
a. Prone position
b. Neutral position
c. Sniffing position
d. None of the above

86. CPT is performed on an 80-year-old woman with pneumonia. She has a history of chronic obstructive pulmonary disease, osteoporosis, and diabetes. Breath sounds include rales bilaterally and minimally productive strong cough. She is alert and oriented, and is able to cough and deep breathe upon command. Which of the following actions is most appropriate to take in this situation?
a. Perform the CPT per the physician's order.
b. Change the patient to positive expiratory pressure (PEP) therapy as tolerated.
c. Discontinue CPT.
d. Perform both B and C.

87. A 17-year-old boy is admitted for cystic fibrosis. He is taking 2.5 mg albuterol nebulizer treatments every 8 hours, budesonide 0.5 mg treatments twice daily, and vest therapy twice daily. It is time for all three of this patient's therapies. Which of the following choices describes the best sequence of therapy?

    a. Vest therapy, albuterol, budesonide
    b. Albuterol, budesonide, vest therapy
    c. Albuterol administered during vest therapy, and then followed by budesonide
    d. Vest therapy followed by albuterol and budesonide in one hour

88. A 40-year-old woman is being mechanically ventilated in the adult intensive care unit. Her settings are as follows; yesterday: AC, 500, 14, +5, 45% PIP=45, Plat=31, inspiratory flow = 45 L/min. Today: AC, 500, 14, +5, 45% PIP=47, Plat=30, inspiratory flow = 45 L/min. Which of the following is true about this patient's airway resistance?

    a. The airway resistance has increased since yesterday.
    b. The airway resistance has stayed the same since yesterday.
    c. The resistance is unable to be calculated with the information above.
    d. The airway resistance has decreased since yesterday.

89. The blood gas results on the patient in question 88 is as follows: PH 7.33, CO_2 47, PO_2 91, HCO_3 22. Which of the following best describes this blood gas result?

    a. Uncompensated respiratory acidosis
    b. Compensated respiratory acidosis
    c. Uncompensated metabolic acidosis
    d. Uncompensated respiratory alkalosis

90. When performing a capillary blood gas on a baby, which of the following actions would be most helpful in obtaining an adequately sized sample?

    a. Use of warming cream
    b. Squeezing the foot firmly
    c. Downward positioning of the foot
    d. Both A and C

91. A 34-year-old woman is receiving 2.5 mg albuterol nebulizer treatment. The patient's breath sounds are clear diminished with faint expiratory wheezes. Before the treatment begins, her heart rate is 90/min and her respiratory rate is 17/min. During the treatment, the patient feels "jittery" and her hands begin to shake. Her heart rate is now 135/min. What is the most appropriate action to take at this time?

    a. Stop the treatment and notify the nurse and doctor.
    b. Continue the treatment and monitor the patient.
    c. Change the patient's treatment to levalbuterol, 1.25 mg.
    d. Perform both A and C.

92. Tracheostomy care is being performed on a patient with copious secretions. During the procedure, the patient's tracheostomy tube becomes dislodged and falls out. The patient begins to gasp and becomes agitated. The patient's oxygen saturation is 88% and he is diaphoretic and pale. Which of the following actions should be taken at this time?
    a. Try to reinsert the tracheostomy tube through the patient's stoma.
    b. Cover the patient's stoma and ventilate via ambu bag and mask.
    c. Call for help and wait for a physician to reinsert the tracheostomy tube.
    d. Perform both B and C.

93. A ventilator check is being performed on a patient in the adult intensive care unit. Her tube was taped at 23 cm at the lip this morning. At this time her tube is now at 25 cm. Which of the following actions should be taken?
    a. Push the tube further in until it reaches 23 cm.
    b. Deflate the cuff, push the tube in until it reaches 23, reinflate the cuff, confirm with chest x-ray.
    c. Remove the tape before making position changes to the tube, then use fresh tape to resecure the tube.
    d. Perform both B and C.

94. A 15-year-old girl comes to the emergency department with an acute asthma exacerbation. Her breath sounds include inspiratory and expiratory wheezes. Her oxygen saturation on room air is 94%. Her respiratory rate is 24/min, and her heart rate is 100/min. She is currently on heliox 80/20 concentration via non-rebreather mask. The patient is currently on a 2.5 mg albuterol nebulizer treatment bled into the heliox setup. The non-rebreather mask's reservoir bag completely deflates during inspiration. The patient states "I feel like I can't breathe." What should be done next?
    a. Assess the patient for change in respiratory status.
    b. Take the heliox off the patient and get a new setup.
    c. Check for leaks, proper mask fit, and adjust flow rate.
    d. Perform both A and C.

95. A 2-year-old girl comes to the emergency department. The patient's mother states that the patient has had diarrhea and vomiting for the past several days. The patient is pale, lethargic, and irritable. The patient's capillary refill time is delayed. The patient's oxygen saturation is 88%, heart rate is 154/min, and respiratory rate is 38/min. Her blood pressure is within normal limits. Which of the following actions should be taken at this time?
    a. Give the patient a fluid bolus of normal saline 20 mL/kg and place the patient on supplemental oxygen.
    b. Give the patient a fluid bolus of lactated ringers 10mL/kg and place the patient on supplemental oxygen.
    c. Ventilate with ambu bag and mask.
    d. Place patient on continuous pulse oximetry, provide supplemental oxygen, and monitor the patient's respiratory status.

96. The patient in question 95 has been treated, and now has a normalized capillary refill time, normal blood pressure, and is now resting comfortably. Her heart rate is 120/min, respiratory rate is 27/min, and her oxygen saturation on a non-rebreather mask is 100%. What actions should be taken now that the patient's status has changed?

    a. Give another fluid bolus of lactated ringer's 20 mL/kg.

    b. Wean the oxygen as tolerated and monitor for changes in the patient's condition.

    c. Discharge the patient.

    d. Admit the patient to the pediatric intensive care unit and continue the patient's current FIO2.

97. A 14-year-old boy comes to the emergency department with acute bronchitis. The patient states he was in the emergency department 2 days ago. At that time he was administered a 2.5 mg albuterol treatment, to which he responded well. He was given an albuterol inhaler and was sent home. The patient says he was supposed to take 2 puffs of the medication every 4 hours. The patient states the inhaler isn't working for him and he still doesn't feel well. The patient's breath sounds include faint inspiratory and expiratory wheezing with good aeration throughout. The patient's respiratory rate is 22/min and his heart rate is 80/min. The patient's oxygen saturation is 97% on room air. Which of the following choices is most appropriate at this time?

    a. Increase the patient's dose to 4 puffs every 4 hours and send the patient home.

    b. Increase the patient's dose to 4 puffs every 4 hours and admit the patient to the hospital.

    c. Assess the patient's metered dose inhaler technique.

    d. Start the patient on an hour-long continuous nebulizer treatment.

98. A 65-year-old man with a history of chronic obstructive pulmonary disease (COPD) is receiving in-home respiratory care. He states that his COPD has become more bothersome since starting his new maintenance medication. He says his doctor switched him from an ipratropium metered dose inhaler, 2 puffs twice daily with spacer, to tiotropium, 1 capsule daily. The patient states he liked the ipratropium better because he felt he "got more of the medicine." An inspiratory flow meter reveals that his maximum inspiratory flow rate is 27 L/min. Which of the following statements is true regarding this scenario?

    a. The patient's inspiratory flow is adequate and his tiotropium should be continued.

    b. The patient's tiotropium should be discontinued and he should be back on his previous dose of ipratropium.

    c. The patient should be placed on fluticasone and salmeterol 250/50.

    d. None of the above should be performed.

99. A 19-year-old man is admitted for a head injury due to a motor vehicle accident. The patient has subsequently developed pneumonia and CPT has been ordered. Which of the following positions is NOT appropriate for this patient?

    a. Trendelenburg

    b. Prone

    c. Supine

    d. Semi-Fowlers

100. A 13-year-old boy is having his metered dose inhaler (MDI) technique assessed. He shakes the MDI for 15 seconds, places it in his mouth, presses down on the canister, and inhales quickly. He holds his breath for 10 seconds and then lets his breath out slowly. He then repeats the process after 30 seconds. Which of the following modifications needs to be made in this patient's MDI technique?

a. This patient should use a holding chamber.
b. This patient should inhale slowly.
c. This patient should wait one minute between doses.
d. This patient should do all of the above.

Answers and Explanations

1. C: An arterial blood gas is an invasive procedure that is not indicated at this time, since there is no information indicating that this patient has impending ventilator failure. A chest x-ray is appropriate because the patient may have pneumonia or another pulmonary disorder causing a cough. Option B, pulse oximetry, is a fast and effective way to measure the patient's ventilator status. And option D is appropriate because vital signs are the first assessment that should be performed on a patient.

2. B: Pre-term refers to babies born earlier than 37 weeks. Term refers to babies born at 37-41 weeks.

3. B: Respiratory acidosis is defined as a low pH and high CO_2. Option A is incorrect because respiratory alkalosis is defined as pH greater than 7.4 and CO_2 less than 35 mmol/L. Option C is incorrect because metabolic acidosis is defined as PH less than 7.3 and CO_2 less than 17 mmol/L.

4. C: A pulmonary function test on a patient with chronic obstructive pulmonary disease (COPD) would show a scooped-out flow volume loop, which indicates normal lung volumes with low expiratory flow. These findings are consistent with an obstructive lung disease such as COPD.

5. B: Resuscitation begins with "A, B, Cs" (airway, breathing and circulation). Airway is first, and the patient should be ventilated before any other action begins. Compressions follow second. Rigorous rubbing is not indicated at this time, because it was not successful at the beginning of the resuscitation process. No more time should be wasted on stimulation. Option D is incorrect because a pulse oximetry reading is not important since the therapist already knows the patient is in respiratory failure.

6. C: The symptoms of cough, green sputum, fever, and cough are consistent with pneumonia. Options A and D are incorrect because a patient would not have a fever and decreased percussion notes with an exacerbation of emphysema or asthma. Option B is incorrect because none of the patient's symptoms match a diagnosis of pulmonary edema.

7. D: When assessing a patient for the first time, all aspects of their past medical history must be obtained. These include but are not limited to smoking history and current medications. A smoking history could require tobacco cessation information or treatment to be dispensed during her hospital stay, and could also complicate the patient's current illness. In addition, a current medication history must be obtained so that her home medication regimen can be continued in the hospital and evaluated for potential of causing the patient's symptoms.

8. D: When assessing a patient's psychological state, it is important to determine whether or not the patient is alert and oriented. The patient should be asked questions regarding person, place, and time. They should be able to verbalize their name (person), where they

are (place), and what day it is (time). Additionally, the patient should also be asked about the events leading up to this current illness. If the patient can answer all these questions correctly, then this patient is "alert and oriented times four."

9. D: Endotracheal tube placement measures correctly but should be confirmed with a second evaluation method. An endotracheal tube's placement must be evaluated using more than one criterion. Option A is incorrect because while the endotracheal tube measures correctly in the x-ray, every patient's anatomy is different and the tube may be too far in or out. Option B is incorrect because there is no information in the question as to how what size the tube is and if it is appropriate for the patient's size. Option C is incorrect because the lung fields appear equal and clear, which indicates the tube may be in the correct position. There is no definite information that states the tube is not in deep enough.

10. D: The above symptoms are consistent with epiglottitis. A chest x-ray alone is not appropriate, as the patient needs a view of the neck in order to evaluate epiglottitis. A neck radiograph is not enough on its own because the patient is in respiratory distress based on her symptoms, and should be placed on pulse oximetry to further evaluate her respiratory status.

11. B: The patient's symptoms and neck radiograph are consistent with epiglottitis. A patient with epiglottitis will have a neck radiograph showing an enlarged epiglottis, column of air surrounding the epiglottis, and view of a "thumb sign." Asthma is not the correct answer because this disease is not diagnosed via a neck radiograph. An allergic reaction is not correct because we know that this patient's symptoms are consistent with epiglottitis and the neck radiograph confirms that diagnosis. An allergic reaction radiograph may show swelling of the airway as a whole, not of just the epiglottis.

12. D: This patient has low oxygen saturation but the pulse oximeter's waveform is irregular. An irregular waveform is consistent with a faulty finger probe, poor circulation, or cold hands. All of these factors should be evaluated first before a patient is placed on oxygen therapy. Taking the patients pulse and comparing it to the monitor's heart rate reading would determine whether or not the pulse oximeter is working correctly. If the patient's heart rate on the monitor and the patients pulse do not match, the finger probe on the pulse oximeter is not picking up.

13. A: The symptoms of sweating, anxiety, and chest pain are consistent with several arrhythmias, including supraventricular tachycardia (SVT). The EKG rhythm of a narrow QRS and heart rate of 180 is consistent with SVT. Dizziness is also a symptom of SVT.

14. D: This patient is alert, and should not be shocked by either cardioversion or defibrillation unless they become unresponsive. Vagal maneuvers should be performed first, and if they are not successful, then adenosine should be administered.

15. C: This patient may have obstructive sleep apnea based on his weight, snoring, and desaturating at night. IPAP settings should never exceed EPAP settings. IPAP is providing

positive pressure ventilation to the patient during inhalation, while EPAP is providing PEEP during exhalation. Therefore, option B is incorrect. Options A and D are both incorrect because this patient is desaturating and requires supplemental oxygen. Option C is correct because the IPAP does not exceed EPAP and the patient is being provided with supplemental oxygen to manage the periods of desaturation with sleeping.

16. A: Answer A is appropriate because secondhand smoke is an asthma trigger, and until he is able to quit, secondhand smoke must be eliminated in the home. Option B is not correct because it is never appropriate to pit family members against each other. This can cause undue stress among the family, and stress is also an asthma trigger. Option C is not appropriate because pets, especially ones that the patient is allergic to, must not be kept in an asthmatics bedroom. Option D is inappropriate because if a patient is allergic to dogs, he is allergic to all dogs. Hypoallergenic refers to "less allergy" not "no allergy."

17. B: A tension pneumothorax is characterized by a shift of the trachea to the opposite side as the collapsed lung. The patient will also present with mediastinal shift, increased percussion note, hypotension, and tachycardia. This patient is on mechanical ventilation, and there is no information regarding trauma, so options C and D are incorrect. Option A is incorrect because a left tension pneumothorax would have a tracheal shift to the right, not the left.

18. A: The correct way to perform peak flows is to have the patient stand, take the biggest breath they can and blow it out hard and fast into the peak flow meter. Then repeat that process 2 more times, and choose the highest number to report to the physician.

19. C: Peak flow zones are organized based on percentage of personal best or predicted peak flow number. As we do not know what the patient's predicted number is, one would base the zones off of the patient's predicted number. The green zone is 80-100% of predicted. The yellow zone is 79-51% of predicted, and the red zone is 50%-0% of predicted. Since this patient's peak flow number of 150 is at 48% of their predicted, the patient is in the red zone.

20. A: Auto peep refers to pressure that is trapped in the alveoli after exhalation. Auto peep is determined by observing the flow-time curve on the ventilator's graphics screen. If the expiratory flow does not return to baseline (zero) before inhalation resumes, the patient is experiencing auto peep.

21. D: First, to get millimeters of mercury, multiply 29.95 inches by 25.4 to get 760.73 mm Hg. Then calculate the PAO_2 by using the equation $PAO_2 = (PB-PH_2O) FIO_2-PaCO (1.25) = (760.73-47) 0.35-80 (1.25) = (713.73) 0.35 -100 = 149.81$.

22. A: Using the equation $P(A-a)O_2$, plug in the correct PAO_2 and PaO_2 from the explanation of question 21: 149.81-80 = 69.81 mm Hg.

23. B: When a patient is restless and moving, artifact can be displayed on the EKG rhythm

strip. This patient was stable and speaking. In addition, the patient's pulse was 80/min which is not indicative of ventricular tachycardia. Therefore, further inspection is necessary before assuming the patient needed treatment for ventricular tachycardia.

24. D: Pseudomonas is a gram-negative aerobic bacterium. Pseudomonas infections are not limited to the respiratory tract; they can be seen in other parts of the body as well.

25. D: Based on the patient's symptoms of dull percussion note, diminished breath sounds, and the previous diagnosis of congestive heart failure, it is possible that this patient has a pleural effusion. However, more tests need to be performed in order to confirm this diagnosis. Any of the above tests (chest CT, chest X-ray, or ultrasound) would be helpful in this case.
26. D: Several actions can be performed via bronchoscope, and include but are not limited to airway clearance, visual inspection of the airway, and removal of foreign body or tissue.

27. B: A laryngeal mask airway is an endotracheal tube with a mask attached to the end. The mask sits in the patient's pharynx, not externally over the patient's nose and mouth. This airway is most commonly used in emergency and surgery situations. It is not designed for long-term use due to the risk of aspiration. It is an effective form of ventilation.

28. D: Full-face masks are not always appropriate for patients due to the aspiration risk, as well as the fact that this patient is claustrophobic and may not tolerate a full-face mask. Option B is incorrect because nasal masks must be chosen according to the size and structure of the patient's nose and face. Option C is incorrect because patients with claustrophobia can be treated successfully with CPAP, provided that the clinician and patient work together to determine what mask and settings make the patient most comfortable.

29. C: CPAP can be uncomfortable for claustrophobic patients. Clinicians must work with the patient to make the treatment more tolerable. Some ways to achieve this are to choose an appropriately sized mask or prongs, and setting a ramp so that the pressure gradually builds as the patient gets used to the initial pressure setting. Merely telling the patient to calm down is not effective and could actually make the patient more agitated. Performing relaxation and or visualization techniques is a more appropriate choice.

30. A: When calculating the total pressure, look at the PIP which is the total pressure delivered to the patient. Option B is incorrect because this value of 15 is the volume of gas delivered to the patient; also known as delta P. Calculate this value by subtracting the PEEP from the PIP. Delta P is what regulates the patient's tidal volume in pressure control mode. Pressure control is a pressure limited mode, so option C is incorrect. Option D is incorrect because pressure control is a full support mode and it is not spontaneous. An example of a spontaneous mode would be pressure support.

31. B: B is not appropriate in this case because adding extension to the patient's tubing may make the decrease in flow worse. Instead of adding an extension, the therapist should be

removing any extra extensions and then re-check the flow. The therapist should also check the tubing for leaks, holes, or kinks. The therapist should also inspect the humidifier for any cracks or loose connections.

32. D: None of the above statements are true regarding quality control measures. The medical director of the blood gas lab must be actively involved in the quality control protocol and results. CLIA requires quality control measures to be performed at least every 8 hours. And lastly, remediation protocols must be in place in the event that the quality control results are out of range.

33. C: The percent change from an FEV1 of 75% to 90% post-bronchodilator shows that the patient has a positive response to the bronchodilator. The FEF 25-75 also increased more than 12%, which is also consistent with a positive change. The increased FVC, TLC, and RV may indicate air trapping from an obstructive disorder. The decreased respiratory flow, and increased lung volumes are also indicative of an obstructive disorder. Choice B is incorrect because asthma cannot be diagnosed from one PFT alone. While asthma is an obstructive disease, which is consistent with the above findings, this patient may have a different obstructive disease. Option A is incorrect because restrictive disorders are characterized by normal expiratory flow and reduced lung volumes, neither of which is indicated in the above results. And choice D is not correct, because we already know this patient gave maximum effort by noting the increased lung volumes measured in this test.

34. D: A patient with clostridium difficile will be in contact precautions. Contact precautions require caregivers to wear a gown and gloves when caring for a patient. While a caregiver may choose to wear a mask for their own personal protection, this is not a standard requirement of the contact precautions protocol.

35. D: The avian flu is an airborne illness. Therefore, all patients must be placed in airborne isolation. This includes a negative air flow room, and it also requires all health care workers to wear personal protective equipment including a respirator mask, gown, and gloves. Respirator masks must be fit tested and the health care workers must be wearing the appropriate size. Health care workers must always practice good hand hygiene when caring for patients.

36. B: Option A is not correct because this patient has no signs of an adverse reaction. An adverse reaction includes respiratory distress, increase in heart rate over 20%, and other serious reactions such as an allergic response. Option C is not correct because the patient's breath sounds have actually improved from diminished to wheezing. If a patient starts with diminished breath sounds has wheezing after the treatment, the patient has increased aeration of the lungs and the patient's respiratory status has improved. Option D is not correct because the patient has no signs or symptoms of respiratory distress. The patient's vital signs are within normal limits, and the patient's breath sounds have improved since before the treatment.

37. D: A positive outcome includes not only an improvement in the patient's overall

respiratory status and health, but also the patient's own self-identified goals. The patient's personal goals of therapy must be identified, implemented, and achieved. Option C is incorrect because we know from the information above that this patient has COPD. It is very common for a patient with a chronic lung disease like COPD to be on daily respiratory medications and inhalers. Because it is a chronic condition, COPD is not curable and sometimes requires daily medication in order to control the disease and allow the patient to have a better quality of life.

38. A: Risk factors for ventilator-associated pneumonia include but are not limited to extended length of time on ventilator, supine patient position, condensation in ventilator circuit, and breaking of ventilator circuit. Option B is incorrect because the semi-recumbent patient position (head elevated) is a way to minimize ventilator associated pneumonia. Option C is incorrect because semi-recumbent patient position and shortened length of time are ways to minimize ventilator-associated pneumonias.

39. D: All of the above tools are required for a proper extubation. Suction is needed so that the patient's mouth and endotracheal tube can be suctioned prior to extubation. The 10 cc syringe is required for deflation of the endotracheal tube cuff. And supplemental oxygen is needed after extubation takes place.

40. C: The correct steps to extubation are as follows. First, suction both the patients mouth and endotracheal tube in order to prevent aspiration when extubating. Second, deflate the cuff using a 10 cc syringe. Next, ask the patient to take a deep breath in and blow it out while removing the tube, and lastly place the patient on supplemental oxygen as needed. Option A is incorrect because it does not mention suctioning the patient's mouth, which is an important part of the extubation preparation process. Option B is incorrect because it says to deflate the cuff before suctioning, which can cause aspiration of secretions. Option D is incorrect because it does not include suctioning of the mouth, and it also includes a nebulizer treatment even though there is no information that indicates a treatment is necessary.

41. B: Choice A is incorrect because oral steroids, not inhaled steroids, have potentially severe side effects and are only used in short "bursts." Inhaled corticosteroids are very safe and effective in the treatment of respiratory diseases. Inhaled corticosteroids are commonly used for long periods of time. Choice B is the correct answer. Inhaled steroids are used to treat and prevent inflammation in the lungs. Option C is incorrect because inhaled corticosteroids are commonly used in moderate to severe asthma and are a very effective choice in the management of this disease. Option D is not correct because inhaled corticosteroids can be used in pregnant asthmatics. Some inhaled corticosteroids are a pregnancy class B drug, which is considered an appropriate therapy choice for moderate to severe asthmatic mothers.

42. A: The proper technique for nasotracheal suctioning a child is as follows. First, use measured suction and sterile technique. Lubricate the catheter using lubricating jelly before inserting catheter into the patient's nare and apply suction upon removal. Rinse the

catheter with sterile water or saline and repeat in 30-second intervals as tolerated. Discard the catheter and kit after use. Suction catheters and kits must not be reused on the same patient. Using clean suction catheters and kits for every suctioning session is an important infection control measure.

43. C: The patient is a child with croup. The diagnosis of croup is indicated by the tracheal tugging, upper airway stridor, barking cough, hoarseness, and otherwise clear lung sounds. Croup patients commonly have a near normal oxygen saturation, as does this patient. The first choice of treatment, albuterol 2.5 mg, is not appropriate because this patient does not require bronchodilatation. His breath sounds are clear, and albuterol is not effective in treating stridor. An ipratropium nebulizer is not appropriate for this patient because it is also a bronchodilator and is not effective in the treatment of stridor and croup. Choice D in this question is incorrect because racemic epinephrine is commonly used in croup and would be an appropriate choice of therapy for the patient. The third choice, racemic epinephrine, is the correct answer. Racemic epinephrine reduces edema and relaxes the smooth muscle of the airways, which makes it a drug of choice for croup patients.

44. B: Supplemental oxygen delivery is appropriate because this patient has a low O_2 saturation. Albuterol, 2.5 mg, is an appropriate standard dose for nebulizer treatments. It is a bronchodilator which is the first line drug for asthma management. While the patient's symptoms of chest tightness, wheeze, and cough may indicate a possible diagnosis of asthma, this patient states he has never had breathing problems before. Without a definite diagnosis of asthma from a doctor, providing asthma education is inappropriate. In addition, telling the patient he must stop sports is incorrect. Even if this patient did have asthma, the current asthma guidelines encourage exercise and activity in asthmatic patients. And lastly, monitoring the patient and delaying treatment is not appropriate because this patient has a low O_2 sat and is in respiratory distress. Waiting one hour to give a treatment is potentially dangerous.

45. A: This patient is using a fluticasone and salmeterol diskus, which is a combination inhaled steroid and long-acting bronchodilator. Fluticasone and salmeterol comes in a metered dose inhaler form, but this dosage of 500/50 is only available in diskus form. Therefore, because the inhaler is a DPI, choice C is not correct because spacers can't be used with DPIs. The sweet taste that the patient noticed is a normal side effect of this medication. Choice B is not correct because inhaled steroids take up to several weeks for the patient to feel relief, and the medication should be continued until that time before changing to something else.

46. C:. The correct procedure for performing an arterial blood gas on this patient is as follows: identify the patient using 2 forms of identification, place the patient's wrist on a rolled up towel, perform an Allen test, clean the area with alcohol, insert the needle at a 45-degree angle with the bevel up and the head of the needled going toward the patient, remove the needle when the syringe has an adequate sample, put pressure on the puncture site, and cover with a bandage.

47. D: Capnography is a noninvasive way to measure a patient's dead space and exhaled tidal volume. Capnography can be provided for neonatal and pediatric patients, but it is more difficult in that patient population.

48. D: A patient's CO_2 monitor should have an even and uniform wave pattern. If a wave becomes flattened or appears to be a flat line, it is indicative of a self-extubation or disconnection with the ventilator. Option B, hyperventilation, is not correct because hyperventilation often appears as shorter waves closer together.

49. D: When performing a test on a patient, it is always appropriate to explain how long the test will take, what it measures, and what is required of the patient during the test. The clinician should also explain any side effects that might occur during the test, especially if they are bothersome or painful. In this case, if the patient has asthma, the methacholine challenge may cause chest pain and shortness of breath about which the patient should be warned. Option A is incorrect because warning a patient about side effects will not produce false values on the test. If a patient is not warned of bronchospasm and it does in fact occur, then the patient may panic and cause poor test results.

50. D: This patient has symptoms of asthma including nighttime coughing and wheezing, and shortness of breath upon exertion or exposure to animals. However, due to her previously normal pulmonary function test, she was not diagnosed with asthma by her primary care physician. Bronchoprovocation testing is often ordered to confirm a diagnosis of asthma in a patient who has symptoms of asthma, but also has a history of normal pulmonary function testing. If a bronchoprovocation test like a methacholine challenge shows a positive result, then the diagnosis can be confirmed. This patient had a decrease in FEV1 of 22%. A minimum 20% drop in FEV1 after administration of methacholine is indicative of a positive response to the provocation. And as a result, the patient's diagnosis of asthma can be confirmed.

51. C: This patient's symptoms indicate that the patient is in respiratory distress. The ventilator alarming "high pressure" is consistent with an airway or ventilator obstruction. The ventilator and patient should be carefully evaluated to determine where the obstruction is coming from. In addition, the patient should first be removed from mechanical ventilation and manually ventilated before further investigation can occur.

52. A: The patient's blood gas values show a decreased CO_2 and increased PH, which is consistent with respiratory alkalosis. This patient is 5'7" and weighs 250 lbs. The patient's ideal bodyweight according to his height is 180 lbs. His tidal volume should be 8-10 per kg of his ideal bodyweight of 180 lbs. His tidal volume should be between 648 and 810. His current tidal volume is 900, which is too high according to his ideal bodyweight. Therefore his tidal volume should be decreased in order to normalize his blood gas values and bring his CO_2 back up to normal range.

53. D: When weaning a patient from the ventilator, complete weaning parameters must be performed and measured. Weaning parameters include negative inspiratory force, vital

capacity, and rapid shallow breathing index.

54. B: The average male patient should be intubated with a size 8-9 ET tube. This patient was intubated with a size 7, which is much too small for a patient of this size. The tube should be removed and the patient should be reintubated with a larger ET tube. Option A in incorrect because bagging harder and faster can cause barotrauma and hyperventilation. Option C is incorrect because leaks do not improve spontaneously. Option D is incorrect because pushing more cc's of air into the endotracheal tube cuff can blow the cuff and make the tube unusable.

55. A: This patient has orthopnea, or trouble breathing while lying flat. The best way to alleviate orthopnea is to have the patient sleep elevated on 2 or more pillows at night. Option B, taking a cough suppressant, is not appropriate because the patient does not have any symptoms of coughing. Option C is incorrect because orthopnea may be common in asthma, but it does have treatment options that may alleviate the symptoms for the child. Option D is incorrect because this patient has no symptoms of wheezing, and an inhaler alone will not stop orthopnea.

56. D: Auto peep can be lowered or eliminated by adjusting the set peep to match the auto peep calculated value. Other ways to lower auto peep are to lower the set frequency and lower the set tidal volume. These two adjustments can increase the expiratory time, which will reduce auto peep by allowing the patient more time to exhale. This will reduce air trapping and auto peep.

57. B: This patient has increased pulmonary secretions as indicated by rhonchi, productive cough, and diagnosis of pneumonia. The patient also stated that he felt he was unable to cough up his secretions. Due to these symptoms, the most appropriate action at this time is to add PEP therapy to the patient's regimen for increased secretion mobilization. Decreasing treatments is not appropriate because the patient has wheezing despite nebulizer treatments being administered throughout the day. Option B is incorrect because nasotracheal suctioning should never be performed on alert and oriented patients due to discomfort associated with the therapy.

58. B: The patient's NIF of -23 is adequate for weaning. A NIF must be -20 in 20 seconds in order to support weaning. The patient's VC is 4.9, which is normal for his size. A patient's vital capacity is approximately 20 ml per kg. This patient's weight in kg is 70. So dividing his VC by his ideal bodyweight gives 70 ml/kg, which is a normal vital capacity range for a patient of this size. His RSBI of 95 is also appropriate for weaning because RSBIs must be less than or equal to 105 in order to begin weaning. Option C is incorrect because length of time on the ventilator has nothing to do with weaning as long as the patient has met all other weaning criteria.

59. A: Decreasing a patient's tidal volume will reduce the chances of hyperinflation of the alveoli. Hyperinflation and over distension both contribute to high plateau pressures and subsequent barotrauma. Option B, increasing the tidal volume, would make plateau

pressures rise by adding to the problem of hyperinflation. Option C, increasing the FIO2, would have no effect on the plateau pressure.

60. B: The patient's diagnosis of congestive heart failure and "wet" coarse breath sounds are consistent with uncontrolled congestive heart failure (CHF) and pulmonary edema. The additional information of decreased urine output is also indicative of CHF. The patient's weight is 110 lbs. Converted to kg, the patient's weight is 50 kg. Multiply the patient's weight in kg by 0.5 mL/hour (normal urine output) and the result is a normal urine output of 25 mL/hour for a patient of this size. However, this patient's measured urine output is only 15 mL. Options A and C are incorrect because these interventions are not successful for pulmonary edema from congestive heart failure. CPT is only useful for coarse or rhonchi breath sounds when secretions are present that need to be mobilized.

61. D: In a baby younger than 30 weeks' gestation, it is essential to administer surfactant as soon as possible. Administration of surfactant in addition to positive pressure ventilation via CPAP is an appropriate way to reduce the incidence of respiratory distress syndrome. Manually ventilating the patient via bag and mask is not a correct choice because this patient is breathing on his or her own at an appropriate rate. Grunting and retractions alone are not indicative of acute respiratory failure that requires manual resuscitation.

62. D: All of these patients qualify for a seasonal flu shot if they choose to accept one. The CDC recommends that all people aged 6 months and above receive a seasonal flu shot.

63. D: None of the above choices are true regarding the pneumococcal conjugate vaccine. This vaccine is recommended for all children under 59 months of age, and adults and older children who have risk factors for the development of pneumonia. If a patient has cold symptoms, they may take the vaccine. However, if they have a fever or signs of a more serious illness, the vaccine is not recommended.

64. D: All of the above choices are important parts of a respiratory assessment protocol. Proper assessment of a patient includes past medical history including what medication is taken at home and when the last dose was taken, and peak flow measurements of pre, post, personal best, and predicted. Additionally, cough, oxygen saturation, breath sounds, and chest x-ray are all required of a respiratory protocol.

65. A: When evaluating a patient to determine which drug interventions to order, one must always ask if the patient takes home medications, when the last dose was given, and if the patient has any drug or food allergies. Some inhalers and nebulizer treatments have food derivatives in the medication that can cause allergic reactions if the patient is allergic to that particular food. Option B is not correct because information on food allergies is not enough to form a treatment plan. Option C, while interesting to know, does not determine a pharmacological intervention.

66. B: This patient is allergic to dairy products. Fluticasone and salmeterol diskus has a dairy derivative in the DPI which can cause allergic reactions in patients who are sensitive

to dairy products. Therefore, fluticasone and salmeterol diskus for this patient is contraindicated. However, a fluticasone and salmeterol HFA is appropriate because it does not have the dairy product included in its formula. Option C is not correct because the dosage for that fluticasone and salmeterol HFA is the highest dose possible, which is comparable to the fluticasone and salmeterol 500/50 diskus. The physician wanted this patient on fluticasone and salmeterol 250/50, which is comparable to the fluticasone and salmeterol HFA 115mcg/21mcg with spacer. Option D is not correct because there is no reason why fluticasone and salmeterol would have to be discontinued completely, as there is a more appropriate option in HFA form for this patient.

67. C: This patient takes albuterol treatments every 4 hours and as needed at home. Assuming she was not admitted with any respiratory symptoms, then at a minimum she should have the same drug and frequency of nebulizer treatments ordered as the ones she takes at home. However, since she was in respiratory distress and was taken to the hospital by ambulance, she was given 2 back-to-back nebulizers in the rig. Therefore, we know that her breathing was labored enough to require multiple treatments in a short amount of time. So her current respiratory status of resting comfortably and clear breath sounds are as a result of the previous treatments, and are not a good indicator of her future respiratory status. The best answer is C because this patient requires nebulizer treatments every 4 hours at home, and has required 2 back-to-back just an hour ago. Option A, monitoring the patient for several hours with no further therapy, is incorrect and potentially dangerous. Option B is incorrect because budesonide is an inhaled steroid, is not quick acting, and is not designed to alleviate wheezing. Option D is incorrect because we have no information stating that this patient needs secretion mobilization.

68. D: When educating a patient or family on their medication regimen, it is important to take all of their concerns into account, and alleviate any worries the family has. Telling the mother that all medications have side effects and they will just have to deal with it, is not the best approach when dealing with a mother who is frightened. The best action to take in this situation is to explain that budesonide is not like the bodybuilding steroids, explain the possible side effects and benefits, and tell the mother that this medication is safe and effective for small children.

69. B: The mother has not refused the medication yet, but she is expressing doubts as to the validity of the budesonide's role in her son's medication regimen. Therefore C is not correct, as the mother never formally refused the budesonide. Option A is incorrect because discontinuing the budesonide without any explanation as to why this medication is important, is doing the patient and mother a disservice. In addition, increasing the albuterol to 4 puffs is potentially dangerous because this is twice the recommended dose of this medication. Option B is the correct answer because the mother has stated that she doesn't understand why the budesonide is important, and it is the therapist's responsibility to educate patients and their families on the benefits and risks of all medications prescribed for that patient.

70. A: Intubating a patient is a potentially traumatic event. The patient must have both a

paralytic agent and a sedative in order to keep the patient comfortable. If a patient is only given succinylcholine, the patient is paralyzed but not sedated. Therefore the patient is aware of the entire intubation process including the pain and discomfort associated with that procedure. Combativeness is not a valid reason why this patient can't be intubated, so choice C is incorrect. And D is incorrect because this patient is alert, combative, and coughing. He must be sedated and paralyzed in order to have a successful intubation.

71. B: When performing single-rescuer CPR, the correct compression-to-breath ratio is 30:2, according to the American Heart Association guidelines.

72. A: If an AED is available, it should be placed on the patient immediately. AEDs are an important part of the CPR process because it is designed to quickly analyze and treat rhythm disturbances. If a rescuer waits for one or more rounds of CPR before using the available AED, the rescuer is wasting valuable time. The AED may save the patient's life if used quickly and correctly.

73. D: When transporting a critical patient for over 100 miles, a helicopter has more benefits than ground transportation. However, helicopters also have disadvantages, especially on delicate neonatal patients. Helicopters can be noisy and bumpy during the flight, which can irritate the patient. Altitude-related pressure changes can be bothersome to the patient and require adjustments to ventilation and oxygenation equipment. In addition, helicopters generally have small work areas for patient care on board the aircraft.

74. A: A primary pneumothorax is most common in tall, thin men. We know our patient is a young, healthy man, who is over 6 feet tall, and weighs 180 lbs. Option B is incorrect because secondary pneumothorax is when a pneumothorax occurs as a result of a previous lung disease. This patient has no prior medical history and no other pulmonary symptoms. Option C is not correct because a hemothorax is characterized by blood in the pleural space usually due to some form of blunt trauma. This patient's chest x-ray does not show blood in the pleural space, and the patient was not a victim of trauma. Option D is incorrect because an iatrogenic pneumothorax is most common in a mechanically ventilated patient. Our patient is not being mechanically ventilated at this time.

75. A: When placing a chest tube for a spontaneous pneumothorax in an adult, chest tubes are primarily placed in the fourth or fifth intercostal space in the anterior axillary line.

76. D: The role of the respiratory therapist in a thoracentesis procedure is to monitor the patient, assist the physician, and provide supplemental oxygen as needed. Only a trained physician should perform the invasive thoracentesis procedure of inserting a needle and withdrawing fluid.

77. C: If a patient's home care equipment is broken, the first thing to do is to talk to the patient's case manager. The case manager is responsible for working with the patient's insurance in order to provide the appropriate care and equipment for the patient. Option A, telling the mother that she will have to pay for a new nebulizer, is incorrect. There is no

way to know if the mother has to buy a new one, if the home care company and insurance company have not been contacted yet. Option B is incorrect because the ability of the patient to obtain a new nebulizer has not been evaluated yet. If the patient is not able to obtain a new nebulizer, then adjustments to therapy may need to be made. Option D is not correct because it is never appropriate to take equipment from the hospital and try to make it work on a patient's home care equipment. The parts may not fit or may be faulty, making the hospital liable for any injury that results from this equipment.

78. A: A complete pulmonary function test would be most appropriate for this patient because she doesn't appear to have an active infection, and she may have asthma or another lung disorder that can be diagnosed via pulmonary function testing. A sleep study is not indicated at this time because the patient has symptoms during the day as well as at night. A sleep study alone would not be the best choice for this patient. An arterial blood gas is also not appropriate because it is an invasive and painful procedure that is not indicated at this time.

79. B: Due to the patient's size and symptoms of snoring, daytime sleepiness, headache, and hypertension, the clinician should suspect a diagnosis of obstructive sleep apnea, which can be diagnosed via sleep study. Continuous pulse oximetry monitoring during the day is not appropriate for this patient, as his symptoms are occurring at night. In addition, his oxygen saturation is within normal limits at this time, so further monitoring is not indicated. Arterial blood gas analysis is not indicated at this time due to the patient's normal saturation and absence of respiratory distress.

80. B: When a bipap alarms apnea and low pressure, the cause is either due to a leak in the system, or a change in the patient's condition. The clinician should first assess the patient thoroughly to see if the patient is truly apneic or if there is a leak in the circuit or mask. Option A is incorrect because we do not know yet if the cause is due to the machine or the patient. Turning the alarm limit up is never appropriate without first assessing the patient and determining the patient's respiratory status. Option C is incorrect because the patient has not been assessed and determined to require CPR. An alarm of apnea, does not always match the patient's true respiratory status.

81. A: This patient has extensive trauma to his face, which makes intubation difficult. Attempting a nasal intubation on a patient with extensive nasal trauma is not appropriate. Reattempting oral intubation is not an appropriate choice, as oral intubation has been attempted 3 times previously with no success. In addition, the patient is starting to desaturate and needs a patent airway immediately. Attempting to ventilate via bipap is also incorrect due to this patient's extensive facial trauma. A face mask or nasal mask could cause further damage and/or make ventilation difficult. In this case, an esophageal tracheal combitube would be most appropriate as it is designed to be used for emergency situations and is especially helpful when the vocal chords are not able to be visualized.

82. B: Proper chest wiggle is when the movement is seen on the chest down to the upper thigh. Option A is incorrect because this patient's chest wiggle is not adequate and should

be continuing up to the upper thigh. Option C is incorrect because decreasing the amplitude will decrease her chest wiggle, which is already inadequate. Option D is incorrect because mean airway pressure does not have any direct effect on the chest wiggle.

83. A: Daily quality control measures on a pulmonary function machine include volume calibration and assessment for leaks. Option B, the machine's timekeeping, is measured quarterly. And option C, flow, is measured weekly.

84. D: This patient's peak flow values for the above week were inconsistent. When peak flows are inconsistent and out of range, the patient's peak flow technique should be evaluated and reeducated. In addition, the patient should also be recording and reporting his asthma symptoms during these days. The low values on Wednesday and Thursday should be compared to the patient's symptoms on those days and evaluated for accuracy. Peak flow technique should also be verified with each follow up visit. Option B is incorrect because a predicted peak flow for a patient of this size is approximately 330. A value of 450 is out of range and the respiratory therapist should not assume this is an accurate value.

85. B: Intubating a patient with a combitube is easiest if the patient is in a neutral position. The sniffing position makes intubation with a combitube more difficult than that of a more neutral head position. A prone position would be the most difficult in intubation, such as the patient is on his or her stomach.

86. D: This patient has a history of osteoporosis, which is a contraindication for CPT. Since this patient is alert and oriented, and able to cough and deep breathe on her own, a pep therapy trial would be appropriate. Discontinuing CPT completely without further assessment would be incorrect. We know this patient has rales bilaterally and is unable to cough up all of her secretions. Alternative therapies such as PEP or vibratory PEP therapy could be beneficial.

87. B: The proper sequence of treatment for this patient is a bronchodilator first (albuterol) followed by the steroid (budesonide), and lastly, vest therapy. Nebulizer treatments should not be given during vest therapy as the vibrations of the vest will prevent maximum deposition of medication in the airways. Vest therapy should always be given after nebulizer treatments. The albuterol dilates the bronchioles allowing for better secretion clearance. Bronchodilators should always be given prior to steroids because the bronchodilator will dilate the airways for better steroid particle deposition.

88. A: First convert inspiratory flow from L/min to L/sec: 45 L/min divided by 60 sec= 0.75 L/sec. Next, calculate the airway resistance for both days using the Raw equation (Raw = [PIP-Pplat]/[V L/sec]). Yesterday, Raw = (45-31)/(0.75) = 18.67. Today, Raw = (47-30)/(0.75) = 22.7. Therefore, the resistance has increased since yesterday.

89. A: Normal pH is 7.35 to 7.45, CO_2 is 35-45, and HCO_3 is 22-26. When the pH and CO_2 are low, the ABG is considered a respiratory acidosis. The pH is not within normal limits, so it is also considered uncompensated. Therefore, the patient's ABG is uncompensated

respiratory acidosis.

90. D: When performing a capillary blood gas on a baby, warming the foot and holding the foot in a downward position both help to ensure adequate blood flow to the area and subsequently provide an adequately sized blood sample. Squeezing the foot to release more blood is never appropriate when performing a capillary gas. Squeezing the foot without allowing the blood to flow naturally can cause false results due to tampering with the blood components normally found in a free flowing sample. Gentle "milking" of the foot is acceptable, but squeezing is not.

91. A: This patient's heart rate increased from 90/min to 126/min, which is a 40% increase. If the patient's heart rate increases more than 20%, the treatment should be terminated and the medical staff should be notified. Option B is incorrect because this patient's heart rate has already increased to 40%. Allowing the treatment to continue and potentially increase the heart rate further could be dangerous to the patient. Changing the treatment to levalbuterol, 1.25 mg, is incorrect because this dosage of levalbuterol has the same cardiovascular side effects as 2.5 mg of albuterol.

92. D: When a patient's tracheostomy tube becomes dislodged or falls out, the patient's respiratory status must be evaluated. If the patient is not in respiratory distress, the clinician can attempt to reinsert the tracheostomy tube on their own. However, we can see from his agitation, paleness, desaturation, and diaphoresis that the patient is in respiratory distress. When a patient is in respiratory distress, the clinician must ventilate the patient with a bag and mask while covering the stoma.

93. D: Choice A is incorrect because simply pushing the tube further into the trachea can cause damage from the cuff rubbing against the trachea. The best practice is to remove the tape, deflate the cuff, reposition the tube to the original position, reinflate the cuff, and retape with fresh tape. The therapist would then confirm the tube placement with a chest x-ray.

94. D: When a patient feels dyspneic, the first thing that the clinician needs to do is to assess the patient for change in respiratory status. In this situation, we know that the non-rebreather mask's reservoir bag completely deflates during inspiration, which means that there could be a leak, faulty valves, or lack of adequate flow. Therefore, the clinician should assess the patient and then check for leaks, mask fit, and flow rate. Option B is incorrect because it is possible to fix the heliox setup without having to remove it and find a new setup. This would also cause a time delay in the patient's treatment.

95. A: This patient is in compensated hypovolemic shock, which is categorized by an increased capillary refill time, tachycardia, tachypnea, and normal blood pressure. The cause of the shock is most likely the patient's history of vomiting and diarrhea. The patient also has a low oxygen saturation, which requires treatment. Therefore the best treatment at this time is to place the patient on supplemental oxygen and give the patient a fluid bolus of 20 mL/kg. Option B is incorrect because while lactated ringers is an appropriate choice,

the dose is not correct. The lactated ringer's fluid bolus dose for hypovolemic shock is 20 mL/kg. Option C is incorrect because this patient is breathing adequately. Option D is incorrect because this patient has delayed capillary refill time and therefore needs to increase her fluid intake immediately. Providing oxygen and monitoring devices alone could be potentially dangerous because we are not treating the hypovolemic shock.

96. B: This patient's status has changed and the patient now has normalized capillary refill time and her vital signs are within normal limits. The best action to take at this time is to wean her oxygen as tolerated and monitor the patient for changes in her condition. Option A, giving another fluid bolus, is incorrect because since the patient's capillary refill time has normalized, she no longer needs fluid boluses to increase her blood volume. Option C is incorrect because while the patient is more stable, she is still on 100% oxygen and requires further monitoring. Option D is incorrect because her saturation is 100% on 100% oxygen via non-rebreather. Oxygen should be weaned whenever possible.

97. C: We know albuterol has alleviated the patient's symptoms during his last emergency department visit. However, the patient states that the nebulizer worked for him but the inhaler didn't. Since the nebulizer and MDI were ordered at the same dosage, the metered dose inhaler (MDI) should have brought the patient relief. Therefore, the clinician should assess the patient's MDI technique before increasing the dosage or changing the treatment plan. Option A is incorrect because the patient's dose is being increased to two times the standard dose of albuterol. In addition, the patient is being sent home without being assessed in his MDI technique. If the patient is using the inhaler incorrectly, he may need more education in order for him to get the full benefit of this medication. Option B is incorrect because the dosage is double the standard dose of albuterol and the patient is not showing signs of respiratory distress or complications that would require hospitalization. Option C is incorrect because the patient has good aeration and mild wheezing, which is not an indication for a continuous nebulizer treatment.

98. B: This patient's inspiratory flow rate is only 27 L/min. The minimum inspiratory flow rate for DPIs is 30 L/min. Therefore options A and C are incorrect. This patient does not have adequate inspiratory flow for the proper deposition of the tiotropium. In addition, the patient states that ipratropium worked well for him in the past. Therefore, discontinuing the tiotropium and changing the patient back to ipratropium is appropriate.

99. A: When a patient has a head injury and is at increased risk for elevated intracranial pressure, the Trendelenburg position must be avoided. Placing the patient's head lower than his body can increase intracranial pressure. This action may be dangerous for a patient with a head injury. The prone, supine, or semi-Fowlers positions can all be implemented into the patient's CPT as tolerated.

100. D: Holding chambers are recommended for patients of all ages because they help to slow down the MDI inhalation process, and allows for better deposition of the drug in the patient's airways. The patient's MDI technique does require some adjustments in order for this patient to get the full benefit from his MDI. This patient is breathing in too quickly

when inhaling the MDI dose. Patients should push firmly on the canister and breathe in slowly for the best particle deposition. The manufacturer of albuterol HFA also recommends that patients wait at least one minute in between doses.

Special Report: Study Guides Which Are Worth Your Time

We believe the following practice tests and guide present uncommon value to our customers who wish to "really study" for the test. While our manual teaches some valuable tricks and tips that no one else covers, learning the basic coursework tested on the exam is also necessary.

Respiratory Care Exam Review: Review for the Entry Level and Advanced Exams (Book with CD-ROM)

http://www.amazon.com/exec/obidos/tg/detail/-/072168288X/qid=1091030606/sr=8-3/ref=sr_8_xs_ap_i3_xgl14/102-8498963-0118557?v=glance&s=books&n=507846

Entry Level Respiratory Therapist Exam Guide (Book with CD-ROM)

http://www.amazon.com/exec/obidos/tg/detail/-/0323007392/qid=1091030606/sr=8-2/ref=sr_8_xs_ap_i2_xgl14/102-8498963-0118557?v=glance&s=books&n=507846

Master Guide for Passing the Respiratory Care Credentialing Exams (4th Edition)

http://www.amazon.com/exec/obidos/tg/detail/-/0130138320/qid=1091030606/sr=8-7/ref=sr_8_xs_ap_i7_xgl14/102-8498963-0118557?v=glance&s=books&n=507846

These guides are THE best comprehensive coursework guides to the licensure exams. If you want to spend a couple months in preparation to squeeze every last drop out of your score, buy these books!

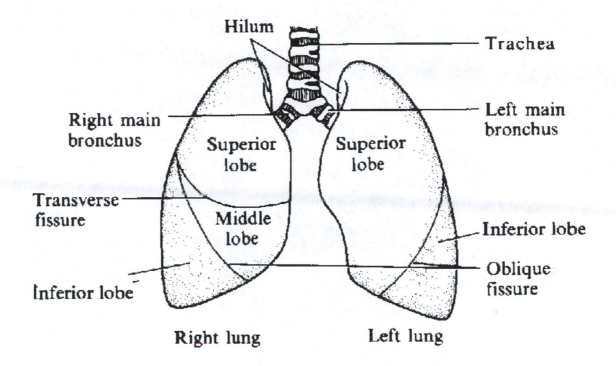

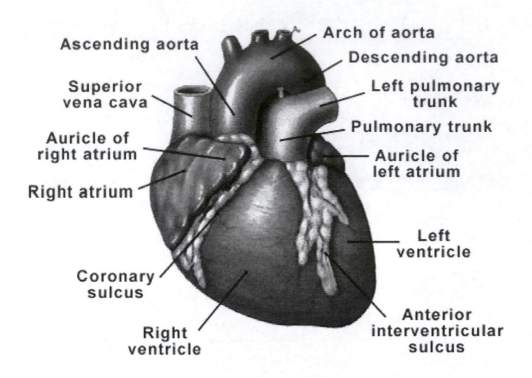

Ascending aorta

Arch of aorta

Descending aorta

Superior
vena cava

Left pulmonary
trunk

Pulmonary trunk

Auricle of
right atrium

Auricle of
left atrium

Right atrium

Left
ventricle

Coronary
sulcus

Right
ventricle

Anterior
interventricular
sulcus

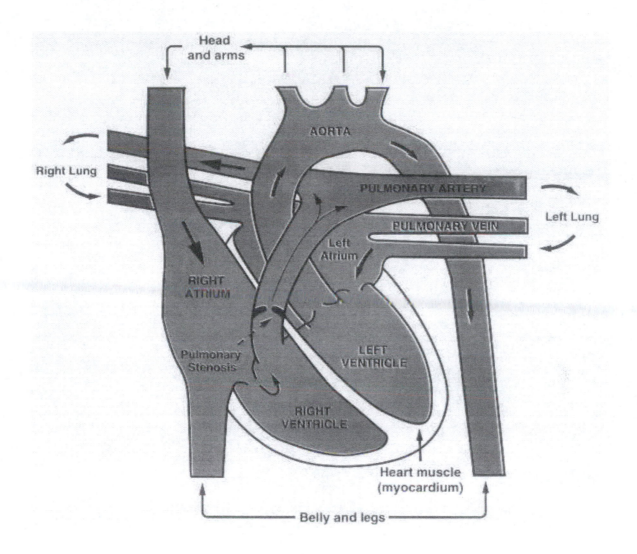

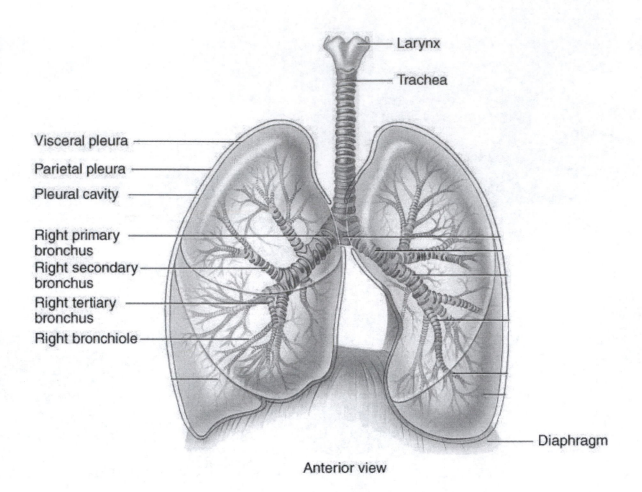

Larynx

Trachea

Visceral pleura

Parietal pleura

Pleural cavity

Right primary bronchus

Right secondary bronchus

Right tertiary bronchus

Right bronchiole

Diaphragm

Anterior view

Special Report: Normal Lab Values

Hematologic

Bleeding time (template)	Less than 10 minutes
Erythrocyte count	4.2-5.9 million/cu mm
Erythrocyte sedimentation rate (Westergren)	Male: 0-15 mm/hr; female: 0-20 mm/hr
Hematocrit, blood	Male: 42-50%; female: 40-48%
Hemoglobin, blood	Male: 13-16 g/dL; female: 12-15 g/dL
Leukocyte count and differential	Leukocyte count: 4000-11,000/cu mm; 50-70% segmented neutrophils; 0-5% band forms, 0-3% eosinophils, 0-1% basophils, 30-45% lymphocytes, 0-6% monocytes
Mean corpuscular volume	86-98 fL
Prothrombin time, plasma	11-13 seconds
Partial thromboplastin time (activated)	30-40 seconds
Platelet count	150,000-300,000/cu mm
Reticulocyte count	0.5-1.5% of red cells

Whole blood, Plasma, serum chemistries

Amylase, serum	25-125 U/L
Arterial studies, blood (patient breathing room air)	
PO2	75-100 mm Hg
PCO2	38-42 mm Hg
Bicarbonate	23-26 mEq/L
pH	7.38-7.44

Oxygen saturation	95% or greater
Bicarbonate, serum	23-28 mEq/L

Bilirubin, serum:

Total	0.3-1.0 mg/dL
Direct	0.1-0.3 mg/dL

Comprehensive metabolic panel:

Bilirubin, serum (total)	0.3-1.0 mg/dL
Calcium, serum	Male: 9.0-10.5 mg/dL; female: 8.5-10.2 mg/dL
Cholesterol, serum (total)	Desirable: less than 200 mg/dL
	Borderline-high: 200-239 mg/dL (may be high in the presence of coronary artery disease or other risk factors)
	High: greater than 239 mg/dL
Creatinine, serum	0.7-1.5 mg/dL
Glucose, plasma	Normal (fasting): 70-115 mg/dL
	Borderline: 115-140 mg/dL
	Abnormal: greater than 140 mg/dL
Phosphorus, serum	3.0-4.5 mg/dL

Proteins, serum:

Pre-Albumin	.2 - 0.4 g/dL
Albumin	3.5-5.5 g/dL
Urea nitrogen, blood (BUN)	8-20 mg/dL
Uric acid, serum	3.0-7.0 mg/dL
Calcium, serum	Male: 9.0-10.5 mg/dL: female: 8.5-10.2 mg/dL
Chloride, serum	98-106 mEq/L

Cholesterol, serum:	Desirable: less than 200 mg/dL
Total	Borderline-high: 200-239 mg/dL (may be high in the presence of coronary artery disease or other risk factors)
	High: greater than 239 mg/dL
High-density lipoprotein	Low: less than 40 mg/dL
Low-density lipoprotein	Optimal: less than 100 mg/dL
	Near-optimal: 100-129 mg/dL
	Borderline-high: 130-159 mg/dL (may be high in the presence of coronary artery disease or other risk factors)
	High: 160-189 mg/dL
	Very high: 190 mg/dL and above
Creatinine, serum	0.7-1.5 mg/dL
Electrolytes, serum:	
Sodium	136-145 mEq/L
Potassium	3.5-5.0 mEq/L
Chloride	98-106 mEq/L
Bicarbonate	23-28 mEq/L
Follicle-stimulating hormone, serum	Adult male: 2-18 mLU/mL
	Female: 5-20 mLU/mL (follicular or luteal)
	30-50 mLU/mL (mid-cycle peak)
	greater than 50 mLU/mL (postmenopausal)
Glucose, plasma	Normal (fasting): 70-115 mg/dL
	Borderline: 115-140 mg/dL
	Abnormal: greater than 140 mg/dL

Lactate dehydrogenase, serum	140-280 U/L
Osmolality, serum	280-300 mOsm/kg H2O
Oxygen saturation, arterial blood	95% or greater
Phosphatase (alkaline), serum	30-120 U/L
Phosphorus, serum	3.0-4.5 mg/dL
Potassium, serum	3.5-5.0 mEq/L
Proteins, serum:	
Sodium, serum	136-145 mEq/L
Triglycerides, serum (fasting)	Normal: less than 250 mg/dL
	Borderline: 250-500 mg/dL
	Abnormal: greater than 500 mg/dL
Urea nitrogen, blood	8-20 mg/dL
Uric acid. Serum	3.0-7.0 mg/dL

Special Report: Key Formulas

Cardiovascular Values

Cardiovascular Values		
Parameter	Derivation	Normal Range
MAP (Mean Artery Pressure)	diastolic + [systolic - diastolic]/3	80-95 mmHg
Pulse Pressure	[systolic – diastolic]	30-50 mmHg
SaO_2 (Arterial Oxygen Saturation)	measured, pulse ox	95-100%
SvO_2 (Mixed Venous Oxygen Saturation)	measured	60-80%
PaO_2 (Partial Pressure of Oxygen - Arterial Blood, Arterial Oxygen Tension)	measured (ABG), [100 - (age - 25)/3]	78-100 mmHg
$PaCO_2$ (Partial Pressure of CO_2 - Arterial Blood, Arterial CO_2 Tension)	measured (ABG)	35-45 mmHg
RAP (Right Atrial Pressure), CVP (Central Venous Pressure)	measured	2-10 mmHg
RVP (Right Ventricle)	measured	15-30 / 0-5 mmHg
PAS / PAD (Pulmonary Artery Systolic / Pulmonary Artery Diastolic) = PAP (Pulmonary Artery Pressure)	measured	15-30 / 8-15 mmHg

PCWP (Pulmonary Capillary Wedge Pressure), PAOP (Pulmonary Artery Occlusion Pressure)	measured	5-16 mmHg
SVR (Systolic Vascular Resistance)	$[(MAP - CVP) \times 79.9] / CO$	770-1500 dynes-sec/cm^5
SVRI (Systolic Vascular Resistance Index)	$[(MAP - CVP) \times 79.9] / CI$	1950-2450 dynes-sec/cm^5/m^2
PVR (Pulmonary Vascular Resistance)	$[(MPAP - PAOP) \times 79.9] / CO$	20-150 dynes-sec/cm^5
PVRI (Pulmonary Vascular Resistance Index)	$[(MPAP - PAOP) \times 79.9] / CI$	50-280 dynes-sec/cm^5/m^2
SV (Stroke Volume)	CO / HR	55-100 ml/beat
SVI (Stroke Volume Index)	CI / HR, or SV / BSA	35-60 ml/beat/m^2
LVSW (Left Ventricular Stroke Work)	SV x (MAP – CVP) x 0.0136	60-105 g-m/beat
LVSWI (Left Ventricular Stroke Work Index)	SVI x (MAP – CVP) x 0.0136	42-62 g-m/m^2/beat
RVSWI (Right Ventricular Stroke Work Index)	SVI x (MPAP – PAOP) x 0.0136	12-17 g-m/m^2/beat
RVEDV (Right Ventricular End Diastolic Volume)	SV / EF	100-150 ml
CaO$_2$ (Arterial O$_2$ Content)	$[(Hb \times 1.34)\, SaO_2] + [PaO_2 \times 0.0031]$	16-22 ml O$_2$ / dl blood
CvO$_2$ (Mixed Venous O$_2$ Content, where v = mixed	$[(Hb \times 1.34)\, SvO_2] + [PvO_2 \times 0.0031]$	12-17 ml O$_2$ / dl blood

venous)		
$C(a-v)O_2$, or $AVDO_2$ (AV O_2 Difference)	$CaO_2 - CvO_2 = (Hb \times 1.34) \times (SaO_2 - SvO_2)$	3.5-5.5 ml O_2 / dl blood
CO, Q_t, (Cardiac Output) – Fick Equation, where V = consumption	$SV \times HR =$ $VO_2 / [C(a-v)O_2 \times 10]$	4-8 l/min
CI (Cardiac Index)	CO / BSA	2.8-4.0 l/min/m^2
DO_2 (O_2 Delivery)	$CaO_2 \times CO \times 10$	700-1400 ml/min
DO_2I (O_2 Delivery Index)	$CaO_2 \times CI \times 10$	600-800 ml/min/m^2
VO_2 (O_2 Consumption)	$C(a-v)O_2 \times CO \times 10$	180-280 ml/min
VCO_2 (CO_2 Production)		150-230 ml/min
OUC, O_2ER (Oxygen Utilization Coefficient, Oxygen Extraction Ratio)	VO_2 / DO_2	0.23-0.32
RQ (Respiratory Quotient)	VCO_2 / VO_2, where $VCO_2 = CO_2$ production	normal: 0.75-0.90 pure carbohydrates: 1.0 protein: 0.8 fat: 0.7
CcO_2 (Pulmonary End Capillary O_2 Content)	$(Hb \times 1.37 \times 1) + 0.0031 [0.5(P_{ATM} - 47) - P_ACO_2]$	
Q_s / Q_t (Shunt Fraction)	$[CcO_2 - CaO_2] / [CcO_2 - CvO_2]$	0.05, or 5%

Respiratory Values

Respiratory Values

Parameter	Derivation	Normal Range
TLC (Total Lung Capacity)	$TLC = VC + RV$	80 ml/kg, or about 5.0-6.0 liters
VC (Vital Capacity)	$VC = IRV + ERV + TV$	> 75-80% predicted
V_E (Minute Ventilation)	$TV \times RR$	4-6.5 l/min, or about 100 ml/kg/min
P_AO_2 (Alveolar O_2 Pressure, Alveolar Air Equation)	$(P_B - P_{H2O})FiO_2 - [PaCO_2 \times 1.25]$, where $P_B = 760$ mmHg at sea level, and $P_{H2O} = 47$ mmHg, and 1.25 is the inverse of the RQ	
PaO_2 (Arterial O_2 Pressure)	measured	room air: 80-100 mmHg
A-a Gradient (Alveolar Arterial Oxygen Gradient)	$P_AO_2 - PaO_2 = [(713) FiO_2 - PaCO_2 \times 1.25] - PaO_2$	room air (21% FiO_2): 2-22 mmHg; 100% FiO_2: 10-60 mmHg
Oxygen Index	PaO_2 / FiO_2	500
VA (Alveolar Ventilation)	$[VCO_2 / PaCO_2] K$	4-6 l/min
VD / VT (VD = dead space, and VT = tidal volume) – Bohr Equation* or Physiologic~	$*[P_ACO_2 - P_ECO_2] / P_ACO_2$, or $\sim[P_aCO_2 - P_ECO_2] / P_aCO_2$	0.2-0.4
R_{aw} (Airway Resistance)	$[P_{alv} - P_{mouth}] / V$	1.5-2.0 cm H_2O/l/sec
Compliance	*delta* Volume / *delta* Pressure	
Static Compliance	VT / [Plateau Pressure – PEEP]	50-85 ml/cm H_2O

Dynamic Compliance	VT / [Peak Inspiratory Pressure – PEEP]	75-125 ml/cm H_2O
Chest Wall Compliance	VT / [Airway Pressure – Intrapleural Pressure]	
Pulmonary Blood Flow Distribution	Zone 1: $P_A > P_a > P_v$ Zone 2: $P_a > P_A > P_v$ Zone 3: $P_a > P_v > P_A$	

Acid/Base Relationships

Anion Gap	$Na^+ - (Cl + HCO_3)$, with normal range 8-12 mmol/l or mEq/l
Base or Bicarbonate Deficit, Metabolic Acidosis (mEq/l)	0.4 (wt in kg) x [desired bicarbonate – observed bicarbonate]
Free Water Deficit	(0.6) x (wt in kg) x [(serum sodium / 140) - 1]; Note - measured in liters, fluid Rx for hypernatremia, infuse 50% of calculated deficit over 1st 24 hours and the remainder over the following 1-2 days
Henderson Hasselbach Equation	$pH = pK + \log[(HCO_3) / (H_2CO_3)]$, or $pH = 6.1 + \log[(HCO_3 / 0.03 (PaCO_2)]$
Hydrogen Ion Concentration	$[H^+]$ nm/l = 24 (PCO_2) / HCO_3
Rules for Metabolic Compensations for Primary Acute and Chronic Respiratory and Alkalosis	1. During acute hypercapnia, HCO_3 increases 1 mmol/l for each 10 mmHg increase in $PaCO_2$ above 40 mmHg. 2. During chronic hypercapnia, HCO_3 increases 3-4 mmol/l for each 10 mmHg increase in $PaCO_2$ above 40 mmHg.

	3. During acute hypocapnia, HCO_3 decreases 2 mmol/l for every 10 mmHg decrease in $PaCO_2$ below 40 mmHg. 4. During chronic hypocapnia, HCO_3 decreases 4-5 mmol/l for every 10 mmHg decrease in $PaCO_2$ below 40 mmHg.
Oxyhemoglobin Dissociation Curve and Alkalosis (alkalosis shifts the curve to the left)	Each 0.10 pH rise lowers the PaO_2 about 10%, and oxygen availability to tissues is also reduced by about 10% for each pH increase of 0.10.
Osmolality, Calculated	$[2 \times Na^+]$ + BUN/2.8 + Glucose/18 + ETOH/4.6 + Ethylene Glycol/6.2 + Methanol/3.2 + Isopropanol/6.0
Osmolar Gap	Measured Osmolality – Calculated Osmolality; An osmolar gap > 10 mOsm/l suggests the presence of abnormal solutes such as lactate, methanol, ethanol…
pH Changes	1. If the pH rises by 0.10, then K^+ falls an average of 0.5 mEq/l. 2. If the pH rises by 0.10, then ionized calcium and magnesium fall 3-8%.
Parkland Formula (Burn Resuscitation)	4 ml crystalloid / kg / % burn - over 24 hours (50% over the first 8 hours, then 50% over the following 16 hours)
Sodium Bicarbonate Replacement Dose	(base deficit in mEq/l) x (wt in kg) / 4; Note - replace 1/2 of the deficit over 8-12 hours in a non cardiac arrest situation.
Winter's Formula, Respiratory Compensation for Metabolic Acidosis	$PCO_2 = (HCO_3)(1.5) + 8 \pm 4$

Pediatric Considerations

Blood Pressure - Systolic, age 1-10, 50th percentile	90 mmHg + (age in years x 2) mmHg
Blood Pressure - Systolic, lower limits, 5th percentile	70 mmHg + (age in years x 2) mmHg
Creatinine Clearance	[0.48 x ht in cm x BSA] / [creatinine in mg/dl x 1.73]
Defibrillation for Ventricular Fibrillation or Pulseless Ventricular Tachycardia	2 J/kg, then 4 J/kg, then 4 J/kg
ET (Endotracheal) Tube Size (internal diameter - mm)	(16 + age in years) / 4, or [(age in years) / 4] + 4; Note - use an uncuffed ET tube for ages < 8 years.
ET (Endotracheal) Tube Insertion Depth Determination	12 + (age in years / 2) cm; Note - measured from lips.
Fluid Deficit Replacement	[(estimated deficit - %) / 100] x (wt - kg); Note - give 1st half over the first eight hours, and the 2nd half over the next 16 hours.
IV Continuous Infusions	[6 x dose (ug/kg/min) x wt in kg] / rate (ml/hr) = mg of drug / 100 ml fluid

Secret Key #1 - Time is Your Greatest Enemy

Pace Yourself

Wear a watch. At the beginning of the test, check the time (or start a chronometer on your watch to count the minutes), and check the time after every few questions to make sure you are "on schedule."

If you are forced to speed up, do it efficiently. Usually one or more answer choices can be eliminated without too much difficulty. Above all, don't panic. Don't speed up and just begin guessing at random choices. By pacing yourself, and continually monitoring your progress against your watch, you will always know exactly how far ahead or behind you are with your available time. If you find that you are one minute behind on the test, don't skip one question without spending any time on it, just to catch back up. Take 15 fewer seconds on the next four questions, and after four questions you'll have caught back up. Once you catch back up, you can continue working each problem at your normal pace.

Furthermore, don't dwell on the problems that you were rushed on. If a problem was taking up too much time and you made a hurried guess, it must be difficult. The difficult questions are the ones you are most likely to miss anyway, so it isn't a big loss. It is better to end with more time than you need than to run out of time.

Lastly, sometimes it is beneficial to slow down if you are constantly getting ahead of time. You are always more likely to catch a careless mistake by working more slowly than quickly, and among very high-scoring test takers (those who are likely to have lots of time left over), careless errors affect the score more than mastery of material.

Secret Key #2 - Guessing is not Guesswork

You probably know that guessing is a good idea - unlike other standardized tests, there is no penalty for getting a wrong answer. Even if you have no idea about a question, you still have a 20-25% chance of getting it right.

Most test takers do not understand the impact that proper guessing can have on their score. Unless you score extremely high, guessing will significantly contribute to your final score.

Monkeys Take the Test

What most test takers don't realize is that to insure that 20-25% chance, you have to guess randomly. If you put 20 monkeys in a room to take this test, assuming they answered once per question and behaved themselves, on average they would get 20-25% of the questions correct. Put 20 test takers in the room, and the average will be much lower among guessed questions. Why?

1. The test writers intentionally writes deceptive answer choices that "look" right. A test taker has no idea about a question, so picks the "best looking" answer, which is often wrong. The monkey has no idea what looks good and what doesn't, so will consistently be lucky about 20-25% of the time.

2. Test takers will eliminate answer choices from the guessing pool based on a hunch or intuition. Simple but correct answers often get excluded, leaving a 0% chance of being correct. The monkey has no clue, and often gets lucky with the best choice.

This is why the process of elimination endorsed by most test courses is flawed and detrimental to your performance- test takers don't guess, they make an ignorant stab in the dark that is usually worse than random.

$5 Challenge

Let me introduce one of the most valuable ideas of this course- the $5 challenge:

You only mark your "best guess" if you are willing to bet $5 on it.

You only eliminate choices from guessing if you are willing to bet $5 on it.

Why $5? Five dollars is an amount of money that is small yet not insignificant, and can really add up fast (20 questions could cost you $100). Likewise, each answer choice on one question of the test will have a small impact on your overall score, but it can really add up to a lot of points in the end.

The process of elimination IS valuable. The following shows your chance of guessing it right:

If you eliminate wrong answer choices until only this many answer choices remain:	1	2	3
Chance of getting it correct:	100%	50%	33%

However, if you accidentally eliminate the right answer or go on a hunch for an incorrect answer, your chances drop dramatically: to 0%. By guessing among all the answer choices, you are GUARANTEED to have a shot at the right answer.

That's why the $5 test is so valuable- if you give up the advantage and safety of a pure guess, it had better be worth the risk.

What we still haven't covered is how to be sure that whatever guess you make is truly random. Here's the easiest way:

Always pick the first answer choice among those remaining.

Such a technique means that you have decided, **before you see a single test question**, exactly how you are going to guess- and since the order of choices tells you nothing about which one is correct, this guessing technique is perfectly random.

This section is not meant to scare you away from making educated guesses or eliminating choices- you just need to define when a choice is worth eliminating. The $5 test, along with a pre-defined random guessing strategy, is the best way to make sure you reap all of the benefits of guessing.

Secret Key #3 - Practice Smarter, Not Harder

Many test takers delay the test preparation process because they dread the awful amounts of practice time they think necessary to succeed on the test. We have refined an effective method that will take you only a fraction of the time.

There are a number of "obstacles" in your way to succeed. Among these are answering questions, finishing in time, and mastering test-taking strategies. All must be executed on the day of the test at peak performance, or your score will suffer. The test is a mental marathon that has a large impact on your future.

Just like a marathon runner, it is important to work your way up to the full challenge. So first you just worry about questions, and then time, and finally strategy:

Success Strategy

1. Find a good source for practice tests.
2. If you are willing to make a larger time investment, consider using more than one study guide- often the different approaches of multiple authors will help you "get" difficult concepts.
3. Take a practice test with no time constraints, with all study helps "open book." Take your time with questions and focus on applying strategies.
4. Take a practice test with time constraints, with all guides "open book."
5. Take a final practice test with no open material and time limits

If you have time to take more practice tests, just repeat step 5. By gradually exposing yourself to the full rigors of the test environment, you will condition your mind to the stress of test day and maximize your success.

Secret Key #4 - **Prepare, Don't Procrastinate**

Let me state an obvious fact: if you take the test three times, you will get three different scores. This is due to the way you feel on test day, the level of preparedness you have, and, despite the test writers' claims to the contrary, some tests WILL be easier for you than others.

Since your future depends so much on your score, you should maximize your chances of success. In order to maximize the likelihood of success, you've got to prepare in advance. This means taking practice tests and spending time learning the information and test taking strategies you will need to succeed.

Never take the test as a "practice" test, expecting that you can just take it again if you need to. Feel free to take sample tests on your own, but when you go to take the official test, be prepared, be focused, and do your best the first time!

Secret Key #5 - Test Yourself

Everyone knows that time is money. There is no need to spend too much of your time or too little of your time preparing for the test. You should only spend as much of your precious time preparing as is necessary for you to get the score you need.

Once you have taken a practice test under real conditions of time constraints, then you will know if you are ready for the test or not.

If you have scored extremely high the first time that you take the practice test, then there is not much point in spending countless hours studying. You are already there.

Benchmark your abilities by retaking practice tests and seeing how much you have improved. Once you score high enough to guarantee success, then you are ready.

If you have scored well below where you need, then knuckle down and begin studying in earnest. Check your improvement regularly through the use of practice tests under real conditions. Above all, don't worry, panic, or give up. The key is perseverance!

Then, when you go to take the test, remain confident and remember how well you did on the practice tests. If you can score high enough on a practice test, then you can do the same on the real thing.

General Strategies

The most important thing you can do is to ignore your fears and jump into the test immediately- do not be overwhelmed by any strange-sounding terms. You have to jump into the test like jumping into a pool- all at once is the easiest way.

Make Predictions

As you read and understand the question, try to guess what the answer will be. Remember that several of the answer choices are wrong, and once you begin reading them, your mind will immediately become cluttered with answer choices designed to throw you off. Your mind is typically the most focused immediately after you have read the question and digested its contents. If you can, try to predict what the correct answer will be. You may be surprised at what you can predict.

Quickly scan the choices and see if your prediction is in the listed answer choices. If it is, then you can be quite confident that you have the right answer. It still won't hurt to check the other answer choices, but most of the time, you've got it!

Answer the Question

It may seem obvious to only pick answer choices that answer the question, but the test writers can create some excellent answer choices that are wrong. Don't pick an answer just because it sounds right, or you believe it to be true. It MUST answer the question. Once you've made your selection, always go back and check it against the question and make sure that you didn't misread the question, and the answer choice does answer the question posed.

Benchmark

After you read the first answer choice, decide if you think it sounds correct or not. If it doesn't, move on to the next answer choice. If it does, mentally mark that answer choice.

This doesn't mean that you've definitely selected it as your answer choice, it just means that it's the best you've seen thus far. Go ahead and read the next choice. If the next choice is worse than the one you've already selected, keep going to the next answer choice. If the next choice is better than the choice you've already selected, mentally mark the new answer choice as your best guess.

The first answer choice that you select becomes your standard. Every other answer choice must be benchmarked against that standard. That choice is correct until proven otherwise by another answer choice beating it out. Once you've decided that no other answer choice seems as good, do one final check to ensure that your answer choice answers the question posed.

Valid Information

Don't discount any of the information provided in the question. Every piece of information may be necessary to determine the correct answer. None of the information in the question is there to throw you off (while the answer choices will certainly have information to throw you off). If two seemingly unrelated topics are discussed, don't ignore either. You can be confident there is a relationship, or it wouldn't be included in the question, and you are probably going to have to determine what is that relationship to find the answer.

Avoid "Fact Traps"

Don't get distracted by a choice that is factually true. Your search is for the answer that answers the question. Stay focused and don't fall for an answer that is true but incorrect. Always go back to the question and make sure you're choosing an answer that actually answers the question and is not just a true statement. An answer can be factually correct, but it MUST answer the question asked. Additionally, two answers can both be seemingly correct, so be sure to read all of the answer choices, and make sure that you get the one that BEST answers the question.

Milk the Question

Some of the questions may throw you completely off. They might deal with a subject you have not been exposed to, or one that you haven't reviewed in years. While your lack of knowledge about the subject will be a hindrance, the question itself can give you many clues that will help you find the correct answer. Read the question carefully and look for clues. Watch particularly for adjectives and nouns describing difficult terms or words that you don't recognize. Regardless of if you completely understand a word or not, replacing it with a synonym either provided or one you more familiar with may help you to understand what the questions are asking. Rather than wracking your mind about specific detailed information concerning a difficult term or word, try to use mental substitutes that are easier to understand.

The Trap of Familiarity

Don't just choose a word because you recognize it. On difficult questions, you may not recognize a number of words in the answer choices. The test writers don't put "make-believe" words on the test; so don't think that just because you only recognize all the words in one answer choice means that answer choice must be correct. If you only recognize words in one answer choice, then focus on that one. Is it correct? Try your best to determine if it is correct. If it is, that is great, but if it doesn't, eliminate it. Each word and answer choice you eliminate increases your chances of getting the question correct, even if you then have to guess among the unfamiliar choices.

Eliminate Answers

Eliminate choices as soon as you realize they are wrong. But be careful! Make sure you consider all of the possible answer choices. Just because one appears right, doesn't mean that the next one won't be even better! The test writers will usually put more than one good answer choice for every question, so read all of them. Don't worry if you are stuck between two that seem right. By getting down to just two remaining possible choices, your odds are now 50/50. Rather than wasting too much time, play the odds. You are guessing, but guessing wisely, because you've been able to knock out some of the answer choices that you know are wrong. If you are eliminating choices and realize that the last answer choice you are left with is also obviously wrong, don't panic. Start over and consider each choice again. There may easily be something that you missed the first time and will realize on the second pass.

Tough Questions

If you are stumped on a problem or it appears too hard or too difficult, don't waste time. Move on! Remember though, if you can quickly check for obviously incorrect answer choices, your chances of guessing correctly are greatly improved. Before you completely give up, at least try to knock out a couple of possible answers. Eliminate what you can and then guess at the remaining answer choices before moving on.

Brainstorm

If you get stuck on a difficult question, spend a few seconds quickly brainstorming. Run through the complete list of possible answer choices. Look at each choice and ask yourself, "Could this answer the question satisfactorily?" Go through each answer choice and consider it independently of the other. By systematically going through all possibilities, you may find something that you would otherwise overlook. Remember that when you get stuck, it's important to try to keep moving.

Read Carefully

Understand the problem. Read the question and answer choices carefully. Don't miss the question because you misread the terms. You have plenty of time to read each question thoroughly and make sure you understand what is being asked. Yet a happy medium must be attained, so don't waste too much time. You must read carefully, but efficiently.

Face Value

When in doubt, use common sense. Always accept the situation in the problem at face value. Don't read too much into it. These problems will not require you to make huge leaps of logic. The test writers aren't trying to throw you off with a cheap trick. If you have to go beyond creativity and make a leap of logic in order to have an answer choice answer the question, then you should look at the other answer choices. Don't overcomplicate the problem by creating theoretical relationships or explanations that will warp time or space. These are normal problems rooted in reality. It's just that the applicable relationship or explanation may not be readily apparent and you have to figure things out. Use your common sense to interpret anything that isn't clear.

Prefixes

If you're having trouble with a word in the question or answer choices, try dissecting it. Take advantage of every clue that the word might include. Prefixes and suffixes can be a huge help. Usually they allow you to determine a basic meaning. Pre- means before, post- means after, pro - is positive, de- is negative. From these prefixes and suffixes, you can get an idea of the general meaning of the word and try to put it into context. Beware though of any traps. Just because con is the opposite of pro, doesn't necessarily mean congress is the opposite of progress!

Hedge Phrases

Watch out for critical "hedge" phrases, such as likely, may, can, will often, sometimes, often, almost, mostly, usually, generally, rarely, sometimes. Question writers insert these hedge phrases to cover every possibility. Often an answer choice will be wrong simply because it leaves no room for exception. Avoid answer choices that have definitive words like "exactly," and "always".

Switchback Words

Stay alert for "switchbacks". These are the words and phrases frequently used to alert you to shifts in thought. The most common switchback word is "but". Others include although, however, nevertheless, on the other hand, even though, while, in spite of, despite, regardless of.

New Information

Correct answer choices will rarely have completely new information included. Answer choices typically are straightforward reflections of the material asked about and will directly relate to the question. If a new piece of information is included in an answer choice that doesn't even seem to relate to the topic being asked about, then that answer choice is likely incorrect. All of the information needed to answer the question is usually provided for you, and so you should not have to make guesses that are unsupported or choose answer choices that require unknown information that cannot be reasoned on its own.

Time Management

On technical questions, don't get lost on the technical terms. Don't spend too much time on any one question. If you don't know what a term means, then since you don't have a dictionary, odds are you aren't going to get much further. You should immediately recognize terms as whether or not you know them. If you don't, work with the other clues that you have, the other answer choices and terms provided, but don't waste too much time trying to figure out a difficult term.

Contextual Clues

Look for contextual clues. An answer can be right but not correct. The contextual clues will help you find the answer that is most right and is correct. Understand the context in which a phrase or statement is made. This will help you make important distinctions.

Don't Panic

Panicking will not answer any questions for you. Therefore, it isn't helpful. When you first see the question, if your mind goes blank, take a deep breath. Force yourself to mechanically go through the steps of solving the problem and using the strategies you've learned.

Pace Yourself

Don't get clock fever. It's easy to be overwhelmed when you're looking at a page full of questions, your mind is full of random thoughts and feeling confused, and the clock is ticking down faster than you would like. Calm down and maintain the pace that you have set for yourself. As long as you are on track by monitoring your pace, you are guaranteed to have enough time for yourself. When you get to the last few minutes of the test, it may seem like you won't have enough time left, but if you only have as many questions as you should have left at that point, then you're right on track!

Answer Selection

The best way to pick an answer choice is to eliminate all of those that are wrong, until only one is left and confirm that is the correct answer. Sometimes though, an answer choice may immediately look right. Be careful! Take a second to make sure that the other choices are not equally obvious. Don't make a hasty mistake. There are only two times that you should stop before checking other answers. First is when you are positive that the answer choice you have selected is correct. Second is when time is almost out and you have to make a quick guess!

Check Your Work

Since you will probably not know every term listed and the answer to every question, it is important that you get credit for the ones that you do know. Don't miss any questions through careless mistakes. If at all possible, try to take a second to look back over your answer selection and make sure you've selected the correct answer choice and haven't made a costly careless mistake (such as marking an answer choice that you didn't mean to mark). This quick double check should more than pay for itself in caught mistakes for the time it costs.

Beware of Directly Quoted Answers

Sometimes an answer choice will repeat word for word a portion of the question or reference section. However, beware of such exact duplication – it may be a trap! More than likely, the correct choice will paraphrase or summarize a point, rather than being exactly the same wording.

Slang

Scientific sounding answers are better than slang ones. An answer choice that begins "To compare the outcomes..." is much more likely to be correct than one that begins "Because some people insisted..."

Extreme Statements

Avoid wild answers that throw out highly controversial ideas that are proclaimed as established fact. An answer choice that states the "process should be used in certain situations, if..." is much more likely to be correct than one that states the "process should be discontinued completely." The first is a calm rational statement and doesn't even make a definitive, uncompromising stance, using a hedge word "if" to provide wiggle room, whereas the second choice is a radical idea and far more extreme.

Answer Choice Families

When you have two or more answer choices that are direct opposites or parallels, one of them is usually the correct answer. For instance, if one answer choice states "x increases" and another answer choice states "x decreases" or "y increases," then those two or three answer choices are very similar in construction and fall into the same family of answer choices. A family of answer choices is when two or three answer choices are very similar in construction, and yet often have a directly opposite meaning. Usually the correct answer choice will be in that family of answer choices. The "odd man out" or answer choice that doesn't seem to fit the parallel construction of the other answer choices is more likely to be incorrect.

Special Report: Additional Bonus Material

Due to our efforts to try to keep this book to a manageable length, we've created a link that will give you access to all of your additional bonus material.

Please visit http://www.mometrix.com/bonus948/rrt to access the information.